LIVE LONGER!
SEE BETTER!:
For YOU &
Your Optometrist

By Dr Dorie Erickson, MS, Phd, CNC

**Incredible New Life Extension
CardioRetinometry Revealing
Nutritional Secrets Explained**

**Foreword by Prof S.J.Bush, DOpt PhDhc,
endorsed by
Dr K.Walker, MD, PhD; Dr S.Richer, OD., PhD., FAAO.**

ISBN, 978-1-910162-06-4
**Copyright© by Dorie Erickson
November 2013**

New Generation Publishing
The Old Fire Station
140 Tabernacle Street
London
EC2A 4SD

Published by New Generation Publishing in 2013

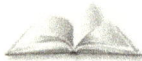

www.newgeneration-publishing.com

New Generation Publishing

Author's note:

As more information became available during the writing of the book, it was decided to compress the lines in parts, rather than expand the pages, thus keeping the book more compact and its cost down, rather than resorting to a smaller type face. Two pages for notes precede the Subject Index

Conflicts of software between the USA writing and the UK writing and editing, resulted in some compromises and amusing errors. Hopefully – we have learned for future collaborations.

Cover Design
Rosalinde Terrill Graphics
Bainbridge Island, WA USA

1

Disclaimer

The information in this book is for educational purposes only and is not intended to diagnose, treat or cure any disease. If you have a medical problem please see your health care professional for guidance as to treatment. It is meant to complement the advice of your health care provider, not to replace it.

It is just as much your responsibility to inform your doctor as it is his or her responsibility to advise you of treatment. Each case is individual with different health backgrounds family histories and present conditions. Thank you.

Table of Contents

Tribute

I wish to pay tribute to Dr Sydney Bush, DOpt., PhD, who inspired me. Without him, this course for CardioRetinometry® would not have been possible as described herein. I also pay tribute to Dr. Ray Hedahl, Optometrist, Poulsbo, WA, USA, who cooperated with Dr Bush in treating my vision needs through the use and transmission of photographs of my eyes as well as his expertise in monitoring my vision for the last twenty years. He has always shown respect for the health choices I have made in eye care and was always willing to help with my vision challenges.

In addition I'd like to honor Dr Linus Pauling to whom we owe much for his unequalled contributions to science and health. Also I honor Dr Matthias Rath, MD and others, including Toronto's gynaecology surgeon philanthropist, Dr Kenneth Walker MD, PhD, also of international journalistic fame (as syndicated columnist W. Gifford-Jones MD) who's acclaim was Dr Bush's great encouragement along the pathway when so many were trying to stop his research.

Dorie Erickson, PhD

Foreword

I am the fourth of five UK generations of Optometrists (a national record) and the first to be extremely proud of having been struck off the register in the defence of Public Health against corrupt Official Medicine. There is much to put right!

Optometrists need Nutritionists! We are both dismayed by exaggerated and excessive claims targeted at our patients for eye related nutrient benefits. I am sure that if eyeglasses are wrongly e.g., 0.75 weak, in magnifying power or too strong in reducing power, such claims e.g., to 'strengthen the eyes,' can be ridiculous. Only the right prescription can suffice. But only qualified nutritionists (NEVER OPTOMETRISTS!) can persuade patients against their wishful thinking! The book is a valuable guide therefore, for both Optometrists and their public.

Exceptional nutritionist Dr Dorie Erickson, DLitt., PhD., CNC is, without doubt, the most highly qualified nutritionist in the World. I asked the former Chancellor of Triune University if she would fill the gaps and extend Optometrists' knowledge. inadequately dealt with in Optometry Colleges.

Many Optometrists overlook that we are an Orthomolecular profession which is the Nobel Prize winner Linus Pauling's term to describe restoring the balance of natural substances in the blood stream. "Toximolecular," is Dr Bernard Rimland's term describing PharmacoMedical substances, never experienced in Nature by humans.

It is no accident that PharmacoMedicne's advertising makes nutrition sound "quaint" and "old fashioned." Dr Erickson reveals how people (and their physicians!) have been lured into believing Pharmacy has the answers. But it pays billions in compensation for abandoned drugs, e.g., Thalidomide (deformed babies) Biaxin and Vioxx (early death.)

Vitamins, correctly taken, are harmless. In the USA alone, properly prescribed drugs in hospitals kill over 100,000 annually and damage over 1,000,000 every year. (Lazorou, Pomeranz, Corey, 2001).
From the American Poison Control Center since 1983 comes this statistic. For Average Deaths Per Year:
  FDA Approved Prescription Drugs 100,000+*
  Non Prescription Drugs – OTC Drugs- 320
  Vitamins, Minerals, Amino Acids – 3
  Herbs – 0. (* Lazarou, Pomeranz & Corey))
  Merck fought hard to keep Vioxx but it caused death and heart attacks; Other examples were Baycol (Cerivastatin deaths) cough medicines (admitted in 2012 in the UK as useless) and Aspirin was found to actually *cause* the coronary heart disease it was meant to prevent! All these and many more, of which people are unaware, have devastating effects. A quick glance at "The PDR. Pocket Guide to Prescriptions Drugs" will alert one to the dangerous side effects of many of these drugs. Part of the burden of these deaths and complications lies with the public who neither read or educate themselves about the dangers which are clearly placed before them though often in very small print.
  Abandoned also are Diethylstilbesterol (teratongenicity - producing monsters) Phenformin (causing acidosis) Ticrynafen (liver damage) Zimeldine (Guillain Barr syndrome) Phenacetin, a popular pain killer for decades (Cancer causing) Methaqualone (addictive) Nomefensine (fatal hemolytic anemia). So when Dr Erickson suggests treatments reminiscent of a popular TV series e.g., Dr Qiunn, Medicine Woman," that is exactly the same knowledge base used by modern pharmacy seeking derivatives for profitable patents, so often with little success.

Natural substances cannot be patented to make big pharmacological profits and will work 1,000 years from now. So restrictive Codex comes to mind!

Pharmacy has produced some notable and extremely valuable drugs as we all know and Dr Erickson properly recognizes this of course. Furosamide and Bumetanide are examples of diuretics that get the kidneys working again. But how very much better it is, if Dr Erickson's natural herbals work for us, without side effects.

She does me the honor of crediting me with far more knowledge of the subject than that which I possess. Gradually increasing and pharmaceutically inspired and supported medical antagonism to the subject of nutrition and vitamins, has been so effective since Szent-Györgyi isolated vitamin C around 1930. We have all suffered. Hard to believe, is the fact that the physicians and pharmacists themselves and their loved ones, have all suffered as a result of medical disinterest at best, sheer obscurantism and even untruths at worst.

In a letter to Dr. Pauling which Szent-Györgyi gave permission to publish, the 1937 Nobel Prizewinner stated that one could take any amount of vitamin C without the least harm. Since then the physicians have pretended that milligrams are sufficient knowing that Hickey & Roberts found over 100 mistakes in the "genocidal" vitamin C RDA evaluation. The USA is more honest than the UK, suggesting four times as much as the criminally inadequate 50 mgs in England, but still gives laboratory primates ten times as much! The truth is that before CardioRetinometry® we didn't know how much vitamin C anyone needed. As Szent-Györgyi says, "we do not know what full health is." But now CardioRetinometry® shows how it varies massively between genders, individuals and how, the need in the same person might escalate with aging. Bruises on the hands of the elderly are a tell-tale sign when there are no teeth to brush, to cause bleeding gums.

The constitution of the World Health Organisation (before predictably taken over and corrupted) says

> "The highest attainable standard of health is one of the fundamental rights of every human being without regard to race, religion, political belief and economic or social condition."

The hidden blockages of the arteries cut life short, introduce disease, and are welcomed by pharmacy and those same corrupt elements in medicine. They see these tenets as intolerably counterproductive to their incomes and actively seek to prevent Optometrists teaching people how to achieve optimal health. Much effort goes into carefully fabricated and publicised disinformation.

We suspect that newspaper editors gain huge sums for allowing ghost writing of articles by the pharmaceutical industry and, similarly, the suppression of good news about vitamins C and E which is so sparse as to be laughable.

The Codex Alimentarius is a wicked instrument pharmacy schemed for over twenty years to introduce. Now it is as good as law everywhere, limiting vitamin strengths without reason, except to boost PharmacoMedical profits. It claims to guarantee "harmonisation!" Vitamin C is then priced beyond reach. The world becomes a more dangerous place every day as pharmacy's enormous wealth corrupts governments and media. Eventually vitamins will only be available on prescription like vitamin C in Germany at perhaps $1/gram!

Overdosing is extremely rare, so pharmacy wins with fewer adverse reactions and more diseases!

So the media play the pharmacy game. Their biggest customer sets the rules. Even the BBC is corrupt .

The record shows how news of CardioRetinometry® has been banned from the BBC and newspapers. Even the pharmacy beholden Optometry journals suppress news about vitamin C in general and the vitamin C encyclopaedia in particular.

How can the supposedly independent non-commercial BBC refuse to review it or interview me again? I told the controller of Northern programmes, after he refused to allow me to be interviewed again, that the BBC had become corrupt, before Saville proved it. Producers have great power.

Another example is the honest study that was carefully carried out by Dr. James Enstrom. PhD. He found that, based on a representative sample of 11,348 non-institutionalized U.S. adults age 25-74 years, who were nutritionally examined during 1971-1974, and followed up for mortality with 1,809 deaths) through 1984, the men gained six and a half years life extension. The statins do not claim even 6 months! More seem to die of cancer, liver, kidney, amnesia, and heart muscle complications. All the time, physicians are trained to play down vitamin C. Now we have the damning evidence!

With no significant benefits from statins imitating it, despite the claims, Pharmacy distorts the picture and encourages people to believe that only the less well informed or 'health freaks' can have faith in vitamin C, and even in vitamin E.

Physicians are trained in making vitamin C a joke. I know because for 3 years, I was there! They say – set a thief to catch a thief! I learned the tricks.

A breakthrough came with the discovery in 1999-that apparently well nourished people could be suffering increasing retinal arterial disease until they started taking extra vitamin C. Astonishingly, amounts needed could vary from none at all for some fortunate folk merely perhaps, needing more sleep, up to massive amounts of well over ten grams.

Then Dr Russell Jaffe MD., JD., in a study, found that some cells needed over 100 grams. My experience showed that many had to have natural vitamin E and Dr. Rath's Lysine also.

Medical resistance, which started even before the discovery of the isolated substance in the 1920s, is easy to understand. As an Optometrist I would have had to find some other career if clever nutritionists had found a simple dietary supplement that prevented the need for reading spectacles! Much as I want to benefit humanity and my fellow man - I want to earn a living, and be here for when simple nutrition cannot suffice.

Ideally, if we could prevent most diseases, there would not be enough broken legs to support all the doctors. They would become like firemen, essential to our lives, and in large numbers when disasters strike.

Vitamin C prevents over 50 diseases – but not for ever! Eventually the decline starts and no matter how we try to meet our escalating needs, we find that birth was a fatal disease.

In 1999 intraluminal plaque was deduced to be the source of the newly discovered variability of appearance of the white line along so many blood vessels.

It was not feasible for the reflex to be, as had always been thought, and is still taught, as an 'ensheathment' of the arteries and arterioles. The laws of reflection contradicted this when a better understanding became available to recognise that two dimensional, flat images of the retinal vasculature could be 'read' in 3 dimensions when one properly understood Pauling/Rath theory and the haemodynamics of circulation.

This has never been explained in the textbooks or teaching of Optometrists. but is fundamental and now we teach it. My critics said "You are not a Professor! " I replied – "Well please tell me who else can teach my subject!" Nobody answered!

 Cholesterol initiated intraluminal plaque (inside the tube) was discovered to be predictable in location, measurable in the living eye, and quantifiable in either its growth or disappearance. It is a different kind of cholesterol – a third kind. VLDL cholesterol is unique to Man. 'High' and 'low' cholesterol are   different.   Plaque cholesterol is 'very low density' which shows the other two to be harmless. It is found wherever pressure against the wall of a blood vessel creates a need for reinforcement due to excessive wear in the absence of sufficient vitamin C, Lysine, Proline and Glycine to make collagen.   I only discovered it because, to avoid adenoviral keratitis in my contact lens wearers, I insisted they took vitamin C and was thoroughly familiar with Pauling-Rath theory. The doctors cannot admit they got it so wrong. Vitamin C & Lysine, the 'Detergent' combination against plaque!

How many unnecessary deaths from premature coronary heart disease has the West suffered since Dr. G. C. Willis proved it to be reversible in 1954/57 ? Since the mid 1950s physicians have been trying to convince themselves that they were right about cholesterol, stressing people with costs and fear. They have made increasing wealth from low cholesterol and low fat foods, polyunsaturates, soya flour, medicines to lower blood cholesterol, home testing kits, etc. triggering e.g Osteoporosis via fat and vitamin D3 deficiency.

In the UK this week, newspapers headline about the *UK Children's Low IQ Due to Fast Food!* Dare they not say that margarines and polyunsaturated oils promoted over saturated fats could have been a dreadful mistake? It is exactly what Denham Harman predicted in *Lancet,* Nov. 1957, cautioning the "rush into dietary polyunsaturates to reduce plasma cholesterol," predicting that "the cure could be worse than the disease!" He will wait for ever for his Nobel Prize.

That is criminal treatment of the man who taught his colleagues about free radicals, antioxidants and vitamin C that they didn't learn at medical school! The Darland High School experiment of Dr. Gwilym Roberts increased IQ by 4.5% with more vit. C!

Eventually in the US, people found that vitamin C lowered their cholesterol just as well as statins! But throughout, we had to wait for Pauling and Rath to solve the puzzle. Around 17,000 studies and papers are to be found trying to link cholesterol with heart disease or researching some aspect of it. But it is the very low density cholesterol with what are called 'Lysil receptors' that are critical to retinal atheroma (plaque) formation and elsewhere. Before 1990 they're irrelevant.

These strands blow around in the bloodstream and catch lysil strands attached to the walls of damaged cells lining the arteries. In the eye the veins too, can be seen to have their fair share of this plaque. It becomes hardened and brittle, and builds until it needs its own blood supply from new, fine capillary networks. In scurvy, these are fragile and when they burst – haemorrhage can strip away the embrittled plaque to form thromboses. These block the vessels further along. It is obvious that 'Low Density' alone is not responsible for the death rate from coronary thrombosis any more than ambulances significantly cause death on the roads. It is what makes the cells lining the arteries weaken, and become unstuck, that then requires a watertight 'puncture repair.'

Now we know that the weakness is collagen losing its strength because of occult scurvy, that no physician can see, just by looking at people, or an occasional blood or lingual test. This is the kind of scurvy that probably affects over 80% of people most of the time and sits, unrecognised, in front of every doctor in the West every day. But it shows up like a lighthouse when we 'flicker alternate' precisely superimposable time lapse, 'before and after' retinal photographs!

Not only were physicians wrong, but their teaching exacerbated the problem. That arteriolar reflex is a healthy retinal sign, has been passed on to Optometry students for 100 years. At the UK General Optical Council "Fitness to Practice" hearing which I deliberately provoked to bring this medical corruption to public attention on 18th - 23rd of June 2012 they found me guilty of misconduct and struck me off but not before I exposed the corruption on Day 2. Being retired and forcibly re-registered, I was furious at the smear but proud to have defended Optometry; the first Optometrist in the World to be proud about being struck off in the cause of Public Health!

I proved photographically, denying all possibility of doubt, that the white vessel plaque is neither a 'healthy' sign as their expert witness, an Optometry lecturer insisted - or harmless! The FTP panel had to smile when I finally asked the stubborn lecturer, which of the two pictures, of arterial disease – the

13

'Before,' or the nine years 'After,' he would prefer for his own! I even began to feel sorry for him, when he said it was "like being back at school," his expertise damaged.

Intraluminal plaque that obstructs blood flow through the arteries is quite different from a hypothesized simple reflection from the arterial wall. There is no doubt that lipid can and does, penetrate the arterial wall, and reflect from it. But I submit that what we see, is much more due to the actual obstructions. They serve the purpose of sealing the artery and vein against leakage of water into the wall of the vessel. This would weaken collagen causing aneurysm. It is made of Lipoprotein alpha [Lp(a)] plasma components and minerals like calcium, as first hypothesized by Pauling and Rath.

Because such fine vessels, 0.15 mm in diameter at most, becoming less than a quarter of that, have such thin walls, they are transparent. They remind us of the 'see through' tropical fish in aquaria.

When it was discovered that it was possible to track the changes in what had to be intraluminal plaque, and that this had always been mistaken for a supposedly harmless 'arteriolar reflex' from the walls of the vessels in photographs of the retina, and in retinal images produced since 1900, either by drawing or later, by photography, a serious rethink about prevention became necessary. But this brought the wrath of the medical profession down on me, supported by – to my astonishment – a very high proportion of Optometrists who did not want to become involved.

I had discovered too much too soon! I had forestalled many years and billions of dollars that could have been spent keeping research doctors in useless comfort.

This has been the pattern for too long with esoteric projects earning huge grants, whilst simple vitamin and nutrient research has been suppressed. The corruption is so bad, that since the 1970s "Selective Indexing" as the editor of the Journal of Orthomolecular Medicine puts it, became censorship.

Every two years, application has been made by this properly peer reviewed journal with illustrious contributors, trying to gain recognition and acceptance by the taxpayer funded National Library of Medicine. But the NLM operates to keep the public ignorant of the true, and often very simple causes of disease, and to maintain high medical incomes. The review committee was privately pre-selected by the NLM.

There are no hearings and no public input is allowed. This is extremely effective and is the next layer of obscurantism and suppression on top of the editorial censorship of the term 'scurvy.' Its effect is that in some years, despite hundreds of millions dying of scurvy related diseases, very few papers can be found, usually varying from around 20 to 30 in the 20,000,000! So physicians tell their patients – even fooling themselves it appears – "Scurvy has gone away – nobody gets it here any more!" Then they die of thrombosis!

The result is then, unbelievably, that the physicians, like the past master of my lodge, and very nearly my father, also die of coronary thrombosis, and it continues as the biggest killer! And they lecture US on how to have healthy hearts!

There is thus no possibility whatever of educating either physicians OR Optometrists properly. Official Western Medicine is fighting tooth and nail by censorship and media control, to *prevent* everyone – INCLUDING DOCTORS and particularly the BBC – from learning the truth! The gang running Western Medicine, particularly in the UK must be made to answer.

The physicians all know very well that when engineered heart disease in the community produces a sudden scurvy related, thrombotic threat to life itself in patients, there is an immediate willingness to open cheque books, and to offer any amount of money for a cure, by the very physicians who helped create the disease, poking fun at vitamin C. It is part of the game. The physicians had only to await the opportunity to demonstrate their skill performing a plumber's type of repair on living arteries to reap their rewards. Heart bypass surgeons will continue to make vast incomes but only for as long as they can keep the public ignorant of the fact that they are performing surgery for a very simple, easily reversible, deficiency disease.

I am certain that people are dying of CoEnzyme Q10 inhibition by statins. There are no inquests! Nobody knows when heart failure is due to the lack of spark! Honest physicians are embarrassed. All physicians realise the potential for creating disease for profit. So the temptation to exploit the availability of massive funds (if people could be persuaded that their hearts needed a re-bore) was too great! And the tragedy is that almost everyone thinks they should thank their lucky stars that wonderful surgeons can save them, to enjoy what's left of their fortunes after paying their hospital bills!

Folk even remain grateful when they discover that their hearts need yet another 're-bore,' or stent, to keep a diseased artery open. And so it goes on. Angioplasty (widening arteries) is another favourite, and all because it was the same doctors who denied them the simple prevention, and insisted that surgical tinkering, ignoring the rest of the diseased scorbutic system, was the best prescription for deficiency.

We know that Dr J. C. Paterson was the first to identify scurvy as the culprit. In the early 1940s – yes over 70 years ago - Dr. Paterson found that almost absent vitamin C in the diseased aorta was the probable cause. So when in 1953, another Canadian, Dr G.C. Willis MD., in Montreal, found that with vitamin C he could dissolve the plaque in Guinea pigs (like humans they make no vitamin C) he wasn't surprised. He demonstrated in humans in 1954, that it could be regressed using the first of the heart X-Rays.

Because he couldn't sacrifice humans like Guinea pigs, he had to invent the system of injecting contrast media into the heart to make X-rays show the obstructions. An enforced cover-up which I have been unable to overcome in the Wikipedia, gives the credit for this to Dr. F. Mason Sones MD. Nobody can get it corrected, and I earned a lifetime ban trying to expose medical extortion!

Emphasising how every effort is thus made to keep the knowledge from the public, they even elected a decoy in Dr. F. Mason Sones, for the major discovery of X-ray coronary angiography! As mentioned already, but now the reader will understand how I cannot over-emphasise how deep the corruption goes, another example is the denial of the Nobel Prize to Prof. Denham Harman.

His mistake – like my own - in discovering too much too soon, was to reveal the importance of free radicals. His hypothesis now – as he says – "reduced to practice" - meaning it is no longer a hypothesis but an accepted theory, sets out how vitamin C quenches the free radicals better than anything else. Since that knowledge is a dreadful threat to pharmaceutical and medical profits, it has to be suppressed beginning with denying Prof. Harman the Nobel Prize for the most important discovery in medicine of the 20th Century. That would attract far too much damaging interest to vitamin C. So Prof Harman and I share the same problem.

I must make it clear that heart disease can take other forms, the prevention of which we still know little. I 'blew' my mitral valve and gave myself an atrial fibrillation. That is when the upper chambers beat at a much greater rate and do not squeeze the blood properly into the ventricles. It sounds very nasty and it is. Anybody can suffer that who unwisely allows their blood pressure and weight to rise as they age.

I was stupid and ignorant of the weak link of heart valves, not having studied other forms of heart disease. A kindly cardiology registrar took the time and trouble to show me my heart dysfunction on the ekocardiograph.

I was not happy to see my mitral valve leaking blood back into my lungs. That can be very fatal! All my medical friends advised exercise! I thought – no! That's the last thing a valve needs that is trying to repair itself!

The cardiologists wanted me to have Warfarin and Aspirin (to 'thin' the blood and prevent clotting). I believed in the vitamin C and E to do the same things only better, putting my trust in honest cardiologist Dr. Matthias Rath, and am still here almost completely cured. White dots passing around my field of vision at the beginning, signified platelet aggregation to me. This is the precursor of thrombosis from blood pooling in the malfunctioning heart. I took more vitamins!

We still need cardiologists and cardiothoracic surgeons but I am pleased now that I avoided the cardio-version trick of deliberately damaging a part of the heart that might be firing off wrong electrical signals. It's a personal choice. Every procedure is an experiment!

Those who attempted to keep this knowledge from the public. actually put fuel into the fire and the determination to let the truth be known, i.e., that heart disease could be prevented and reversed.

On 16th April 2004, I encountered problems with attacks by local doctors via the General Optical Council which – incredibly – eventually became the subject of a harassing Fitness to Practice 'trial,' lasting five full days in June 2012. This quite. farcically implied that I was unqualified to make one of the greatest discoveries of the last Century.

It did not stop the committee finding me guilty of misconduct without a single lay complaint and in the face of 200 written testimonies to the happiness of patients having seen reductions of cholesterol in their arteries, and belief that it was linked to their life extension. During that trial – I was able to prove medical lies and obstructionism of my work. A "stitch up" was how it was described by one of my patients.

The corrupt UK National Health Service withheld my contract. There followed financial penalties as well as character assassination to the UK General Optical Council leading to the trial above

I commented that even proving the untruthfulness of at least one witness and the ignorance of others, and even with the support of Prof Erickson traveling from the USA, and the supportive local chairman of the British Medical Association speaking for me, and also practicing with a medical doctor, there was a determination to convict me of misconduct.

British research physicians then announced proposing to 'start' my field of research in front page newspaper headlines giving me no credit for being the first in 1999, with 'Before and After' images going back to 1998. In the meantime Dr Walker was writing as Dr Gifford-Jones, MD in many newspapers and made it clear several times in his columns that Dr. Bush's "historic discovery is worthy of the Nobel Prize."

Always one for being a rebel, I took the difficult path and fought the opposition. Today I am still fighting the medical resistance but now benefiting from the help of more intelligent advisers and experts in their own field like Dr Erickson. Without her help fundamental to educating apathetic UK Optometrists, I would not be writing this.

Everyone will gain from prevention of coronary heart disease. I would probably have given up were it not for her help e.g., writing this book, as I could not, on my own, educate Optometrists.

Indeed, resistance to change from Optometrists in the UK has been very disappointing. In other countries however, The vitamin C Foundation and Dr. Fonorow, Dr. W. Gifford-Jones MD and Dr. Erickson and leading research Optometrist in the USA, Dr. Stuart P. Richer, at the North Chicago Veterans Hospital that provides me with research facilities, all helped strengthen my resolve. Clearly, UK. medicine resents Optometry. Obviously impossible to cover the subject in one small, condensed volume (a larger book exists solely on vitamin E) Dr Erickson has not finished, and wishes this work to be considered as Volume 1, an indicator for further reading. Much exciting work e.g. phagocytosis, the mitochondria (Denham Harman's 'biological clock') and atherolysis, PUFAs, malacoplakia, the role of trace minerals, Pauling/Rath Unified theory and much more remains to be dealt with in further volumes.

It should be noted that every reference in this book to 'occult scurvy' relates to the condition identified for the first time by CardioRetinometry, as resulting in mild long term deficiency causing cardiovascular pathology and, without doubt, accelerated ageing.

Previously hypothesised as being 'chronic subclinical scurvy,' CardioRetinometry demonstrates occult scurvy as widespread, probably affecting "everybody some of the time, and most people most of the time. "

To those who insist on asking what is the "largest" or "smallest" amount needed, I can reply that from zero to 100 grams/day – only CardioRetinometry at any age can show it. After 150 years of Western Medicine, that is the surprising discovery.

Finally even we were surprised to find on counting –over 500 references listed to mentions of vitamin C in the index.

Sydney Bush, Skidby
East Yorkshire England.   Summer 2013

Acknowledgements

Thank you Dr Ray Hedahl, for your diagnosis that sent me on a search to preserve my eyesight.

Thank you Life Extension (USA) and ZeaVision, Inc for your help with my research.

Thank you Miss Beth La Fontaine for sending me to Dr Fonorow for help with this glaucoma diagnosis.

Thank you Dr Owen Fonorow for directing me to Dr Sydney Bush.

Thank you Miss Dottie Beaver for your encouragement and prayer support in writing this book.

Thank you Dr Bush for extending this opportunity to write a book on Nutrition for Optometrists, as well as other individuals who may be threatened with blindness or cardiac failure.

Thank you for your expertise and cooperation with Dr Ray Hedahl in reading my photos and for encouraging me in my quest with glaucoma, CardioRetinometry® and in writing this book.

We recognize Dr Bush for his accomplishments in the discovery and practice of CardioRetinometry® over more than a decade. Carefully documenting all his work, he was refused by those who oversaw cardio care.

His sadness is that Pauling and Rath overlooked the microvasculature of the eye's retina as offering in-vivo proof that they lacked, for their paper, 'A Unified theory of heart disease,' paralleling - as it does- precisely the same changes as are taking place in coronary vessels. Indeed, this had been first noted by Michelson, Morganroth et al, in 1979. Later, in 2004, Tedeschi-Reiner et al confirmed this, finding a tight relationship between retinal arteriolar disease and coronary artery disease. Many have known for a long time that looking into the eye is like looking into the inner conditions of the human body. Now without surgery or cancer provoking X-rays, disease processes can be followed and neutralized.

In the book Dr. Bush provides proof that Western Medicine is criminally suppressing scurvy as a disease requiring public attention. The proof is concrete. It is cast in stone and the embarrassment of the medical profession will be such, when the public learns how they have been deceived and deliberately subject to diseases by medicine organised for pharmaco-medical profits, that public and physicians will for ever remember the exposure and scorn the villainous doctors deserve.

The perpetual mocking and condemnation of vitamin C by those whose livings come from disease, strongly suggest that huge research has been done by physicians and pharmacy into the potential for harm that vitamin C offers to their profits.

If hundreds of secret studies have shown them what others like Dr Klenner curing the worst virus diseases have found without pharmacy funding, it would more than account for their secrecy, the lack of papers on megadoses and injected vitamin C and the virulence of their attacks on vitamin C researchers. It would fully and satisfactorily explain everything including the laughable absence of vitamin C from Health Supplements in newspapers paid to play the pharmacy game at the expense of the public

Blindness, thrombosis, heart failure, stroke and fifty more diseases are thus being imposed on everyone who is "not in the know."

Preface

Born into a long family tradition of healing and nutrition, it was natural for me to lean toward it as a career. 'Prairie Medicine Woman' was how my paternal grandmother was known to many. I learned much from my mother, a graduate Home Economist and Nutritionist.

It was natural for me after high school to go to university with one objective; to update and expand my knowledge as far as it was possible. My dissertation was 'Ten Major Reasons for Death and Disease in America: How to Prevent Them Through Natural Health'. After the hard work of my PhD., I had to think about earning a living and went into the field of education.

This led me down a long pathway after a BA in Education from the University of Colorado; an Honorary Doctorate in Education; a Masters in Music from Triune University as well as an earned PhD in Biblical Studies to fulfill a childhood dream. The BS, MS and PhD in Nutrition were earned at Clayton College of Natural Health and American Holistic College of Nutrition.

Along the way I wrote courses for two different colleges. I started writing and illustrating booklets for a 'Youthful Body' during one teaching assignment. Another one followed during another teaching assignment concerning 'Family Health.' Becoming acquainted with another world renowned nutritionist, Elizabeth Baker, MA, I launched into a full time practice of Clinical Nutrition, while still on another teaching assignment.

Bucking the opposition before natural health became so popular was not easy but I knew I had something that was real, that worked for my own life as well as my family and others who followed my teaching.

Growing up through the Great Depression, I learned to improvise, to endure, to scavenge for food eating mouldy oranges, and to persevere in gaining any goal in life. By the age of nine I had saved nine dollars toward my college fund when the average man's monthly wage was $20 to $30.

On receiving my first degree, my mother said "This is just the beginning Dorie, you will go much further." So with a Diploma in one hand and a baby in the other arm, I began a long journey, hand in hand with my husband.

I was blessed for many years to have this wonderful life partner who was very supportive in all my aspirations, as well as the encouragement of family and friends who believed in me.

Having always been fascinated by the gift of sight, I was upset to learn that the good Lord had willed – for reasons only He knows – that I should start to suffer from Glaucoma. Fortunately for me – it turned out to be a blessing in disguise for through it I met another kindred soul who further encouraged me in my quest for the best health, UK Optometrist, Sydney Bush whose research properly earned him an honorary PhD.

So in a roundabout way, I came to be writing this book. My intention is to educate readers as to what they can do to make their own health as functional as possible. This may require a few lifestyle changes. As drivers, we all now how easy it is to slip into casual, careless and unsafe ways. It is the same with most things. We acquire bad habits. But as we age – those bad habits will assuredly shorten our lives if we take no steps to adapt. What we need is a permanent pattern for the pursuit of good health practices and to make lasting changes that will not be just a flash in the pan. 'Permanent' is a big word, like 'never.' Being sensible in our expectation and knowing how short lived New Year Resolutions are, we should not expect an immediate magic bullet.

Hoping to solve things for once and for all is too much to expect. But I believe the principles to which I adhere have lengthened my own life and now I am the survivor of all my departed siblings who were disinterested.

Share my beliefs and we shall be winners. Pursuing good health should become your passion, adhering always to good practices. Dr. Irwin Stone predicted life extension.

With my new appreciation of Optometry comes my second intention. It is that all optometrists find in these pages, important answers for their patients, who have so many eye and other diseases. As we learn more – we find that degenerative and other conditions can be detectable and even preventable through observation of the eye.

Some of these conditions previously had no hope of a cure. Now it seems that not only can some unexpectedly be reversed, but even better – prevented.

What was formerly a bleak outlook regarding the preservation of their sight, has led to life extension through the eye! Furthermore, the prevention of coronary artery disease, and rejuvenation of the heart arteries, which necessarily follows as physicians agree, bodes for a much better future.

Consequently, it is my hope, that many
such patients will have their sight extended
and restored. As the new science
of CardioRetinometry® develops, they
will come to praise their optometrists
for helping them in ways that neither they,

nor their Optometrists ever dreamed
would one day become possible.

We do not yet know how many eye diseases will yield to a nutritional approach. Some take fifty years to develop? As life expectancy increases, the demography changes. Previously, tuberculosis, pneumonia and cholera killed. Today they may survive these to suffer other diseases!

Mysterious diseases of the eye may be the most likely to be caused by deficiencies. Poisoning and the toxins of infective agents may imitate them. The revered Dr. Frederick Klenner stated that vitamin C detoxifies all known toxins and venoms.

I shall have a stab at predicting that mega doses of vitamin C, especially if the adequacy of the dose is supported by CardioRetinometry® monitoring the health of the arteries, will produce subtle changes in the demography of eye diseases.

The eye diseases I expect to disappear or become less common are as follows. I enter these here to whet your appetite as to nutritional advances that will help your patients as well as their doctors. Used by permission from Dr Bush's encyclopaedia' 700 Vitamin C Secrets.

<u>Macular Degeneration</u>: Public Health Issue: 30% of Americans are affected (Taylor, Dorey and Nowell) and it is the primary cause of new blindness the vast majority being the 'Dry' type.

Almost 90% of the blindness occurs in the 'wet' type – No clear link has been established but a link exists to lower socioeconomic groups suggesting that malnutrition is a factor. Fruit and antioxidants are strongly indicated with – as a fire insurance, lutein and zeaxanthin plus many times daily ascorbate.

This emerging disease is of rapidly increasing importance. My own most successful case – wet type, was restored to 90% vision in black and white after degenerating to the point where she could not see if the chart was switched on.

Glaucoma: Primary Open Angle: Prevented and blindness risk cured if caught early. Physicians are baffled by 'low tension' glaucoma. Without pressure lowering as an option they have little confidence in preventing blindness (Virno et al. Bietti 1966.) After their two Rome University eye clinic studies Bietti hypothesised, following their success, in reducing intraocular pressure *and for the first time ever, its remaining low after cessation of the therapy* (7,500 mgs vitamin C four times/day i.e. 30 grams/day) that it had repaired the trabeculum, the spongy structure through which the continually formed aqueous that inflates the eye, filters out before reaching the Canal of Schlemm.

Bush thus thought it a vascular disease, explaining its disappearance from his Vit C promoting clinic, along with atherosclerosis and 'dry eye.' Virno almost abandoned his trial after Linner (Sweden) found only a very small IOP decrease with 1 gm of vitamin C.

Retrobulbar neuritis: Wherever due to known viruses and bacteria, Preventable. Curable. If associated with mysterious conditions like Multiple Sclerosis it is more doubtful but remissions of MS with ascorbate are well known to occur.

Episcleritis: Preventable, Scorbutic element.

Retinal detachment: where due to vitreoretinal traction and peripheral tearing spontaneously curable.

without Assessment for laser prophylaxis is desirable in every case exception.

Retinal detachment and tortuosity: Where due to vessel tortuosity caused by atherosclerosis leading to blockage of arteriolar flow or venous return, intraretinal stress lines precede the retinal tear with subsequent detachment, the complete aetiology being revealed by sequential retinal images, showing predictability.

Prevention of the tortuosity avoids the traction, then the tearing and detachment. Sudden irreversible blindness due to thrombosis of the central artery or vein of the retina is a concomitant risk until the atherolysis reduces blockages. Thrombosis supports the author's opinion that the arteriolar reflex is from intraluminal plaque, itself the origin of the thrombus.

Serous retinopathy: Probably scorbutic in origin.

Vitreous opacities: Uncertain but probably scorbutic.

Cataract: Newest treatment: Babizhayev MA et al
N-Acetyl Carnosine lubricant eyedrops possess all in one universal antioxidant protective effects of L-Carnosine in aqueous and lipid membrane environments. Aldehyde scavenging, and trans glycation activities inherent to cataracts: A Clinical Study of the new vision saving drug N-Acetylcarnosine eyedrop therapy in a database population of over 50,000 patients. Am. J.Ther. 2009 May 30th.

Cataract prevented/reduced: See: tissue absorption, concentration and saturation. If the concentration of vitamin C present in the retina were to be repeated in all the tissues of the body, the total vitamin C held would be perhaps 70 grams

(2-3 ounces). See: Nocturnal.

Cataract and corrupt medicine: Early in my career I was taken aside by one of the eye surgeons in Hull who told me "Whatever you do, do not find a cure for cataract." I shall not name him.

Retinal ischaemia: Reversible. Preventable. CardioRetinometry has photographic evidence of the reversibility of retinal ischaemia in a ceased smoking vegetarian who refused to take a vitamin C supplement because she didn't believe in it.

See: Retinal infarcts.
Retinitis
Retinopathy of type 2 diabetes.
Blepharitis
Hordeolum
Bacterial and allergic Conjunctivitis
Corneal ulcer

> The last four will always be a risk due to opportunistic infections as our health cannot be perfectly maintained at all times. But they should be less frequent. Vitamin C is also a far better antihistamine for allergic conjunctivitis but can anyone imagine the National Institutes of Health providing research funds when considering the competition between manufacturers to market successful antihistamines?

Leaving Dr. Bush's *700 Vitamins C Secrets*, the third intention is that we should acknowledge and never forget the giant leap in our understanding of coronary artery disease that only came through the dedicated and prescient research of doctors like J.C. Paterson, G.C. Willis, Linus Pauling and Matthias Rath. We all benefit from their work. We can discuss it later.

It is not possible to list all the doctors and their discoveries for which I personally feel indebted. They have all benefited my own life, and therefore deserve extra mention here. Sir William Osler, Father of Modern Medicine, is praised by Dr Kenneth Walker, who writes as Dr Gifford-Jones, MD. This perceptive doctor quickly spotted the work of Dr Linus Pauling and honest cardiologist Dr. Mathias Rath when others denigrated their new approach destined to take profits from surgery to treat deficiency disease.

Equally quick to perceive the implications for a paradigm shift in medicine that can be brought about by Optometry, Dr Walker then flew to England. He had spotted the research of Optometrist, Dr. Sydney Bush, noted for his own unique contribution. Professor Denham Harman has thrilled and healed me with his antioxidants for his free Radical theory. They are all obvious candidates.

But for sheer and still unmatched jaw dropping innovation, the work of physician Dr Fred R. Klenner, curing 59 consecutive Polio cases, and other 'incurable' viral diseases, exceeds everyone else's work and discoveries. Millions have died because his work has been so suppressed.

Brilliant work was also done by Dr. Robert F. Cathcart III of intravenous vitamin C fame, with Dr. Thomas E. Levy sharing the honors through his erudite books.

The tragedy is that Official Western Medicine is literally controlled by greedy villains who are actually managing epidemiological disease for profit. That is a huge allegation but it is true. We are all suffering because of the undue influence of pharmacy on medical schools curricula. The physicians are taught what suits pharmaceutical profits and not public Health.

Sadly the two are totally incompatible. Dr. Bush knows this well for he was there.

Proof is easy! The two best and latest medical text books together have 1,742 pages. Less than 3 pages in all for scurvy and vitamin C! The most important for intravenous injection, life saving sodium ascorbate, rates no mention at all in the index or text of either book, and all the other ascorbates get no mention in *Medical Biochemistry* (Baynes and Diminiczak) and *Guyton and Hall's Medical Physiology*. In all our physicians are given less than 3 pages on vitamin C compared with 350 pages in the encyclopedia 700 Vitamin C Secrets by Dr. Bush with 100 pages about the politics and economics i.e. the death threat to many diseases and pharmaco-medical profits

The concepts or issues taught in this book support the special benefits of Vitamin C in the field of optometry.
In addition, I would like to mention the Ocular Nutrition Society whose founder, Optometrist Dr. Jeffrey Anshel OD., felt a need for further education among optometrists especially in the field of prevention. The Ocular Nutrition Society conducts a forum where eye doctors can exchange views and new findings. Training is also offered by several of the laboratories who sponsor them to increase awareness of nutrition in eye care. I do hope that you greatly enjoy the book and find it of value in your life.
Signed,

Dorie Erickson, PhD, CNC.

Introduction

Professor Bush wishes it to be understood that this work forms part of the course for the professional Doctorate in CardioRetinometry® of the Cosmopolitan University, conducted by the World Institute of Optometry and CardioRetinometry®   as first propounded by Prof. Bush. It is part theory and part practical, closely supervised in the clinical module. Cosmopolitan University, an unaccredited university, and therefore outside State Control, was chosen for its independence from Pharmacy and Medicine which together, have distorted curricula at medical schools. It was essential to avoid being suppressed more than experience has already shown possible.

Only in this way can the entire course be fully under our control and not subject to the whims of other Universities.

It is from my own experience in a surprising diagnosis of Glaucoma during my regular check up, that I became passionate about this subject. That sparked my interest in other eye diseases such as Macular Degeneration, as well other common conditions such as other forms of glaucoma and retinal diseases, that most have considered incurable. It is said that, "Whatever diagnosis you have, you can't change that." This is not true!

I immediately decided to pursue natural help since I have had a serious sensitivity to so many chemical drugs in my health history. All that was offered to me as a help for this increased IOP was eye drops comprised of chemical drugs which I refused, going instead to the research tables to find out how to help myself in the field of Clinical Nutrition which I was obliged to do being a professional. Reading the ingredients in the drops prescribed to me, I knew that they contained two ingredients to which I had previously shown an allergic reaction. I felt I was really walking a tightrope to blindness, not being able to take those drugs, and yet not knowing any serious studies that had brought the IOP into the normal ranges.

On my next visit to my Optometrist, he was very pleased that my eye pressure had decreased from 29 to 18mms Hg. He said, "I have never seen that before. What did you do?" I then shared my experience with him and went (stupidly) away to change my regimen to another system of nutritional help for Glaucoma. On my next visit, my IOP had gone even higher, to 32mms Hg! So I went back to my original findings and my next visit showed even lower IOP. Upon leaving, my Optometrist, Dr Ray Hedahl said, "Keep doing what you are doing." "And don't stop!", he added very emphatically.

A friend who had been diagnosed with normal pressure glaucoma referred me to Dr Fonorow for help with my case. Upon speaking with him, without hesitation he referred me to Dr. Sydney Bush in UK, who had done considerable studies on Glaucoma.

On contacting Dr Bush, I questioned that he was giving more consideration to the heart than to the eyes! "Yes," he said. And from there I learned over the next several months about the scientific discovery he had made concerning eye and heart health being observable through the eye.

The Background and politics of the new science.

I recalled then that as a young person I had been told that an Optometrist could look into one's eyes and deduce much about one's bodily interior health condition. Dr Bush then explained how the correct interpretation of arterial health by both Optometrists and Ophthalmologists had been delayed by 100 years because everybody thought that the 'arteriolar reflex' was a healthy reflection from an 'ensheathment' of the arterial wall and never realized that they were looking directly at the intraluminal plaque, systemic disease!

He himself had not realized this – simply accepting like everyone else, what he was taught and published in the textbooks until one day he saw a disappearance. This puzzled him for a minute until he realised the explanation. Then it was found to be happening with others. He then found that apparently there was a link to how much people took his advice about supplementing with vitamin C in the diet.

Dr Bush had been urging vitamin C on all his contact lens patients for many years to reduce the incidence of contact lens related eye infections in his specialist practice, and was studying the retinal arteries and optic nerve for earlier signs of glaucoma than had ever been found (Nasal shift). Instead, he found intraluminal plaque. That he found this was entirely due to his search for microscopic arterial displacements whilst possessing a sound understanding of Pauling/Rath Unified theory of heart disease. The two came together for him, after his purchase of the latest, most powerful retinal camera capable of demonstrating microscopic movements of vessels – not expecting that he would instead find at first, inexplicable changes in the vessels themselves.

In 2004, Dr Russell Watkins, MD, a UK lecturer in histo-pathology alerted Optometrists and Bush was alerted (via the UK Manchester Optometry forum) that research by Prof T.Y. Wong claimed hypertension as predictable from arterial changes in fundus photographs. Bush then published two letters in June and November 2004, as British Medical Journal Rapid Responses to Wong claiming disease reversal.

Lack of interest by UK Optometrists led to Bush trying to goad them into public spirited action. *They responded by banning him from the Manchester forum!* Bush emphasised that hypertension was avoidable with reversal of arterial disease, being disgusted with his colleagues apathy. American Optometrists welcomed him. Google finds the letters.

It was in May 2003 that Bush was the first to announce that arterial cholesterol was the feature showing changes in the retina. He also claimed in the same letter that vitamin C appeared to be the main cause of this. He then related that to coronary grades of atheroma and clearly agreed that Rath's Lipoprotein alpha (Lp[a]) was the cause of the atheroma, fully supporting the view of Linus Pauling and cardiologist Dr Mathias Rath MD. His 2003 letter (9 May, "Optician") also described the pathomechanism of atherogenesis. His letters were ignored.

From my studies in Clinical Nutrition I was familiar

with Orthomolecular Medicine in regard to Mental Illness as published by Dr Carl C. Pfeiffer, PhD., MD. I was also familiar with Dr Linus Pauling's work in the use of Vitamin C for so many of the disease conditions of mankind. This brilliant scientist, who was the unique recipient of two Nobel Prizes, should be greatly respected even though some in Western medicine are still repeating the little 'one liner' mantra that says, "Vitamin C only causes expensive urine." The closed mind is sad as it affects many, causing much suffering that is totally unnecessary.

My own youngest sister was denied vitamin C by her doctor in the 1930's. Our mother requested it for her ear infection. He laughed my mother to scorn saying 'Well that would not do any more good than turning her bed around in the room.' My sister spent the rest of her life with severely damaged hearing due to double Mastoiditis infection which almost killed her.

Unfortunately, the lack of continuing education of doctors due to suppression of vitamin C in the medical journals produces looks of disbelief when we quote Pauling/ Rath Unified Theory of coronary Heart disease to them. Examples are atheroma genetic counter-measures, and atheroma metabolic countermeasures. Tragically, they do not know that atheroma is the consequential component of the metabolic counter-measure against genetic anascorbaemia, formed from lipoprotein alpha, a very low density cholesterol which is a risk MARKER and NOT the risk FACTOR of which so many speak. By this means the blood forms a reinforcement of blood vessels, a puncture repair from inside. This prevents escape of the aqueous component of plasma into the wall of the vessel which would weaken it to precipitate a swelling and then a burst – the much feared aneurysm seen in the retina as a microaneurysm, particularly in diabetics suffering 'cellular scurvy' and not diabetic at all.

Similarly, the atheromatous genetic countermeasure is the readiness to form atheroma in vessels which have thicker walls than those in vitamin C producing animals.

From this basis we shall continue and hope that you enjoy the ride and get excited about helping mankind with conditions of the eye and cardio vascular system that hitherto have been considered incurable.

Chapter I
General Healthy Lifestyle

Here I have included the four doctors whom everyone should follow if they are going to have health and longevity with a good quality of life. Since this is a text for the prospective Doctor of CardioRetinometry® program in the planning, it is important for all aspirants to this degree to be acquainted with the basics of good health and good health practices.

I- General Healthy Life Styles
The Heart: What is wrong?

When we look at the increase in heart disease, we see a dramatically increased incidence in the 1990's. A very large percentage of true scientists believe that the cause is directly related to faulty nutrition due to soils that have not been managed well. Excessive crop bearing has led to nutritionally depleted soils and the use of chemical fertilizers has combined to reduce the viability of farming.

The vulnerability of the top soil in America to the high winds that are so common of the great Midwestern United States has not helped. This is said to be the Bread Basket of the world. (Empty Harvest by Dr. Bernard Jensen & Mark Anderson)

There are many theories about the increase of heart disease since Herrick's first discovery of coronary thrombosis in 1912. Stress reduces your plasma vitamin C markedly. This is a direct cause of coronary heart disease. All the following have contributed to increased stress in our lives with reductions of our antioxidant status.

Increases have been seen in Cigarette smoking
Cheaper tobacco
Cheaper Hydrogenated oils
Cheaper Polyunsaturated oils
Margarines
Steam engine introduced to plantations
= cheaper compact sugar no longer imported as bulky sugar cane but refined on plantation
Faster shipments making sugar even cheaper
Confectionary expansion (Sugar)
Ice cream (Sugar)
Jam / marmalade (Sugar)
Alcohol cheaper – (Gin)
Cooking with gas – less 'raw' food
Cooking with electricity - less 'raw' food
Gaslight shortens hours of sleep
Electric light shortens hours of sleep
Entertainment shortens hours of sleep
Increased stress due to film / cinemas.
Education – more reading – shortens hours of sleep in a more literate society
Pocket watches – standardized time = stress
Wrist watches – more timekeeping and stress.
Wheeled transport-- thereby reducing exercise.
Internal combustion engine transports more food and cheaper food.
Produce grown in remote areas reaches cities after losing much vitamin C.
Trains increasing travel and stress
Radio increasing stress
Radiowaves' effect on humans?
Introduction of mercury amalgam fillings.
Stress of Wars 1st WW etc

Newspaper distribution creating stress.
Radio news creating stress.
Increasing crime.
Cheaper coal with electricity and better transport
More pollution from cheaper coal.
Increasing use of fertilizers
Increasing range of consumer goods – greed
Reduced public worship
Increased stress due to TV
Increasing rang of pharmaceuticals /analgesics, causing delayed illness/death.
Increased cancer pharmaceuticals /chemicals /foods
Increased diabetes.
Increased adverse reactions
Increasing power of physicians
Increased iatrogenic deaths
Increased fear of cholesterol
Increased fear of saturated fat
Restaurant food (Margarines / polyunsaturated oils)

In addition, heavily processed foods are laced with chemical preservatives, coloring, nitrites, flavorings etc, all incompatible with a healthy body. From Dr. Wiley who was the leader of what we now know as the FDA, we quote, "No food product in our country would have any trace of benzoic acid, sulfurous acid or sulfites...alum or saccharin....

No soft drink would contain caffeine or theobromine. No bleached flour would enter our interstate commerce. Our foods and drugs would be wholly without any harm of adulteration and misbranding. The health of our people would be vastly improved and life greatly extended. The manufacturers of our food supply, and especially the millers, would devote their energies to improving public health and promoting happiness in every home by the production

of whole ground, unbolted cereal flours and meals."
(Poisons in Your Food, June Winters)

Organic food

For many years people interested in health were made objects of derision. In the 1990's people began to understand the message. In 2012 nobody laughs any more at the concept of 'organic' foods. People who were regarded as cranks can now quietly smile and think if not say, "I told you so!"

The 'New' prevention

The same is happening with the learned profession of Optometry. Resistance to the notion that one can actually *see* the impact of nutrition on arteries has found it hard to gain acceptance. Even wise Optometrists took a step back and were plainly discomfited by the idea. Did it reflect on their ability to detect adverse changes? Had it been under their noses making them feel inadequate?

Every Optometrist without exception has to accept that it was so. Every Optometrist without exception, has to accept that there were times when the retinal arteries must have improved as people stopped worrying about money, or started taking supplements in general, or stopped smoking, or perhaps and in particular, started taking vitamin C in seriously larger amounts.

Every Optometrist, Ophthalmologist and Diabetologist has to accept, but not necessarily feel guilty of failing to notice the disappearance at times, of the white line along arteries or at the bifurcations of vessels. It took such a very astonishing, amazing, serendipitous coincidence of circumstances for the discovery to come to light, that one might even think 'Divine Intervention!' It could have taken another fifty years!

American and Canadian Optometrists were quick to accept the discovery. In the UK, Dr Bush found his ideas firmly rejected. The few accepted the concept without question as obvious. Now, when one says "We are what we eat," there is little argument. It is finally accepted.

We are pleased with all the individuals who are out there attempting to purify the food supply in America. It is not protected by the FDA as it once was, but many other groups are lifting the banner for a healthy population. (Empty Harvest, Jensen and Anderson, page 46)

Other adulterations of the food supply have been imposed on the public through vast marketing schemes to bring in the most dollars, selling our nation into a people who can hardly defend themselves. We are experiencing the great fiasco imposed on us by the tobacco companies, with the endorsements of many medical doctors. It is believed by the most outstanding scientists of our day, that these adulterations in our food supply are directly related at least in part, to the number of deaths by heart disease.

CardioRetinometry® reveals that increased arterial disease can be offset by about fifty different factors that all impinge on our antioxidant status. When one says 'Antioxidant Status,' one means principally – physiological, related to dietary (vitamin C containing foods) supplementary vitamin C, lifestyle, sociological and environmental changes!

A century ago, in 1911, Dr. G. Lindsay Johnson MA., MD., FRCS wrote a text book and pocket atlas of the fundus oculi. It showed retinal arteries that were faithfully recorded from life by Arthur Head FZS. Exactly the same arterial disease can be seen in children today.

Their retinal arteries were faithfully recorded as extremely accurately drawn and painted images. They leave no doubt that there was just as much heart disease in 1911 as now. Life expectancy at the time was short, reduced greatly by infectious diseases, many cities still not having proper waste management and good quality water supplies.

Many changes such as refrigeration, cooking and food processing, have impacted food quality. Vitamin C is lost which can be vital to good health.
We know that stress directly reduces plasma vitamin C levels. Animals produce more when stressed. Humans cannot.

Since the vitamin C dependent heart is the most active muscle in the human body, it requires a host of nutrients to keep it beating 24 hours per day in a life span of 70 years for 840 months, 25,567 days, 613,608 hours, 36,816,480 minutes, totaling 2,208,988,800 seconds. (Nautilus) The heart beats 72 times per minute, 4,300 times per hour and more than 100,000 times per day. (Healthy Heart)

Think about its lifelong job. It is an unbelievable organ and demands our utmost care if we are going to live quality lives. As every mechanic, car or boat race driver will attest, the more powerful an engine, the more maintenance it requires. (Your Birthday, Nautilus Press, Page 47) (Privatera., MD)

If you add these vitamin C depleting factors to the sedentary lifestyle and stressful daily living in concrete cities with polluted air, it does not take a genius to connect the information observed with the increase of poor heart health. In addition, the breakdown of the American Family that leaves fathers, mothers and children to fend for themselves, outside the security of the family, and you have created a stress factor that has reduced the level of health in America.

No one is home to oversee proper nutrition. Children come home and eat high fat or sugar snacks; husbands grab a fast food hamburger at noon, mothers eat peanut butter and cracker snacks for lunch - all washed down with soda pop, lattes, or high sugar milk shakes. Vitamin C is absent from all these foods. In Nature, apart from honey, cereals and bee propolis, no food can be found that does not contain vitamin C. Our diet has gone – with farming and civilization – from one extreme to the other.

Even a diet of Guinea Pigs, that are one of the .0001% of creatures that do not make their own vitamin C, would still provide the vitamin C that the animal had eaten! And here is a puzzle. When Williams and Deason were given 120 weanling Guinea Pigs in 1967, they decided to run a study on how they fared with varying amounts of dietary vitamin C.

 They were divided into 8 groups of 15. the final graphs showed a ridge of greater growth which went through all the groups.

Here is a rough approximation to the results they obtained
Growth with high vitamin C (schematic)

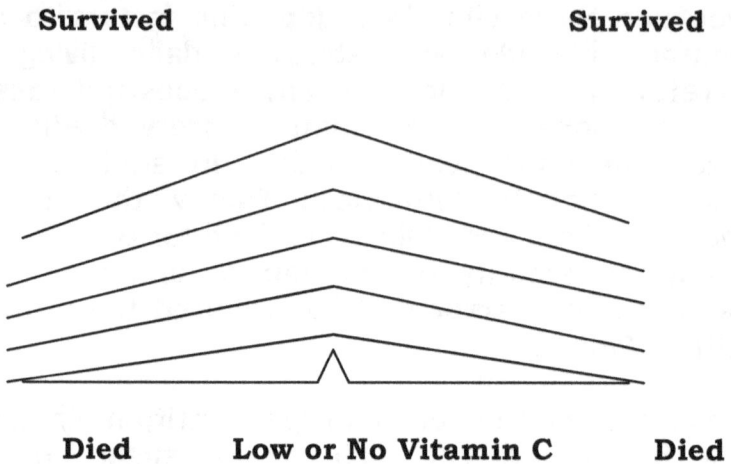

Survived   Survived

Died   Low or No Vitamin C   Died

Guinea Pigs growth given varying dietary vitamin

Guinea Pigs growth given varying dietary vitamin C

The growth patterns showed that in the group receiving NO vitamin C there was one that grew as well as some in the next group above that received some vitamin C.

This graph revealed that not only is there some doubt, about Guinea Pigs, but there must be the same concerns re humans. Do certain individuals, in some mysterious way, make a little vitamin C? In the case of the Guinea Pigs this experiment clearly demonstrated that some individuals exhibited greater and others lower biological need for vitamin C. In all the groups, variations were found at each level of supplementation. Of course this experiment has grave connotations for humans because the majority of people share the inability of the Guinea Pig to make their own.

Also schizophrenics need 10 times more than others. Recent work has changed everything however. It appears from the 1995 work of May, Qu and Whitesell (a hematologist with a sense of humor) that we can regenerate our vitamin C better using our red cells, than other animals. Perhaps most animal experiments now need repeating! 99.9% of animals are compelled to make 1 to100 gms/day!

The Heart: How to Keep it Healthy or Restore its Ability to do its Job.
A healthy heart can be maintained by following simple common sense rules of life.
1) It must have the proper protein nutrition and vitamin C rich foods
2) It must have the right amount of exercise.
3) It must have enough oxygen.
4) Its 8 hr period of repair must be adequate to make good 100% of daily 16 hrs wear and tear.

Most important Heart Supplements
Herbs:

The two most valuable Herbs for the heart are Hawthorne and Cayenne, taken daily. Also, Butcher's Broom a member of the lily family contains two steroid saponins, Lapin and Sannie, which inhibit inflammation in the veins and thus reduce vascular constriction. Another of nature's heart helpers is Rosemary which may be safely used by people of any age and is helpful especially after respiratory or flu type illnesses. (Privitera, Healthy Heart Book p 16)

Crataegus will feed the heart's own circulatory system that it reserves to itself. Avena Sativa will calm the patient so the heartbeat will become normal again.

Cayenne if taken correctly will equalize the heart rate so that it will normalize no matter how fast or slow it is going. That must be done by placing ¼ teaspoon of the hottest Cayenne powder far back on the tongue, then swallowing it with a lot of water. Given in this way the stomach is readied to use it properly rather than just digesting a gelatin capsule and spilling cayenne in the stomach floor.

A very good homeopathic remedy is an extract of the herb Lycopus which opens up the heart, brain and chest cavities relieving a person from pain through all three pathways. (Advanced Treatise in Herbology, Dr Edward E. Shook, p 122)

Vitamins:
The most important Vitamin is Vitamin C from 5,000 mg to 20,000 mg per day. The next important is a Vitamin E that has no chance of turning rancid (Unique E or E Emulsion). Without B6 your heart will still need B6 to convert cysteine to taurine.

Here again, the form of vitamin C most recommended by Dr. Linus Pauling as well as Dr Sydney Bush is Sodium Ascorbate. That is to be increased gradually to bowel tolerance as described by Dr Turska. Vitamin E known for its heart healthy oils comes in 5 different forms. Only two are truly bioavailable.

The first is Unique E
This is because it is all natural as it occurs in nature rather than being humanly engineered or synthetic. It contains all four tocopherol complexes; d-alpha tocopherol, d-beta tocopherol, d-gamma tocopherol and d-delta tocopherol. (Ideally in capsules with glycerol.)

The Second Oil Diluted Mixed Tocopherols.
This form is all natural but does not present it as in nature itself. It comes from soy and although it contains all four tocopherols, it is mixed with other oils that turn rancid even in soft gel caps, giving a huge dose of oxidants, thereby rendering its purpose null and void.
 The other three forms are

3) Synthetic E- d-alpha tocopherol
This form has unwanted side effects such as heart palpitations, and digestive disturbances. It was accepted as an industry standard in 1941. It is used in most all vitamin E studies, rendering them useless. It is extremely important that you do not spend a SHORTER lifetime using this form of vitamin E.

4) Esterified Vitamin E (d-alpha Acetate or Succinate).
This is chemically produced and uses all four forms in an esterified formulation producing only one tocopherol. It resists oxidization and thereby does not act as an antioxidant. Like the synthetic form it does not provide natural vitamin E complex.

5) Tocopherol-Tocotrienol Combination.
Two plant sources from nature are combined, processed together and in so doing result in the cancellation of one or the other of the tocopherols thereby rendering it incomplete. (A.C.Grace Company brochure)

Minerals:

Selenium is the most important mineral.
Calcium, magnesium and potassium are also vital for a healthy heart - or for that matter, any muscle or function that works in a "thrust and relax" repetitive

action such as the heart, bowels, lungs, bladder, etc.

Aminos:

The most valuable Amino Acid for vision and the heart is L-Lysine 800 mg per day. This is contained in red meat and dairy products, so if you are vegetarian you must supplement your diet with Lysine an important amino for heart and vessel health. Taurine, a sulfur amino acid is also needed for heart health as well as cysteine.

L-carnitine helps build muscle endurance and is needed by this important muscle. If you are environmentally conscious and don't want to eat red meats contaminated by chemical fertilizer, pesticides, antibiotics, and hormones you will also have to supplement or find a source of naturally grown beef. Some people feel that they can use wild meats as a protection against these, but I wouldn't count on it due to the diseases carried by wild animals, and the spray residues that they could get in their food.

Homeopathic:

Homeopathy is based similarly to the medical theory of desensitizing a person for allergies by giving something that is offensive (eg. house dust) in minuscule amounts. In the medical model the body then becomes less sensitive to the offending allergen after many injections over a long period of time.

In Homeopathy however, a minuscule amount is given of a substance that will cause the symptom such as flower pollens which causes sneezing. The body then sets up defenses against that invader and sets in process a system of the body itself fighting that condition.

Used for centuries to relieve suffering in both animals and mankind, some still refuse to believe that it works. Veterinary homeopaths can point to identical herds of cows that differ in susceptibility to mastitis only because of the homeopathic remedy dropped into their drinking water. In the human model we can say that improvement took place because the person believed it would help, as in a placebo effect, but for animals, that explanation is invalid.

Foods:
The most important changes in your diet are listed below.
• Under eating but over nutrition: This may be a new concept to most. Dr Walford, MD, *Maximum Lifespan*
• Eat as many raw, fresh, organic foods, as possible. Elizabeth Baker, *The UN Cook Book.*
• No sugar, gluten products, or white flour. Dr Perricone, *The Perricone Prescription.*

Other Factors:
Chondroitin Sulfate A is a mucopolysacharide, a hormone like substance, which is vitally important for heart health and has also been shown to ". . . reduce cancers of the lung, pancreas, ovary, rectum, prostate, cervix and thyroid." (James Pitman. MD. Healthy Heart Book, p 15.)

Exercise:
Importantly, keep vitamin C levels high for your heart to keep your body internally clean so that the bowels are clean and free without causing internal pressure on any organ. Often poor digestion or elimination puts undue pressure on the heart causing frightening angina like pains. In addition, an over fat body also

deposits fat around or in the heart muscle, making an unhealthy heart. Exercise will correct faulty metabolism so you do not have to "starve yourself".

The next thing is enough exercise every day to make your heart muscles strong. This exercise should be gradually increased in length and difficulty until your heart is beating at a maximum for your age and condition. To challenge cardiovascular conditioning a strict schedule should be adhered to and if you already have a heart condition you should work in conjunction with your health care professional. "Your maximum heart rate is calculated by subtracting your age from 220."

I find this chart, from Cathy Smith's Walkfit for a Better Body, very helpful and it takes away the mystery of it all. The idea is to start where you are and build the strength of that heart. If you have any existing heart condition you should be under the guidance of your health care professional, so that you gain heart strength, rather than hurting yourself.

Maximum heart rate.
For example if you are age 40, your maximum heart rate is approximately 180. Take 60% of 180 (108) for the low end, and 80% (which is 144) for the high end. Then try to walk at a pace that keeps your heart rate above 108, but below 144.

This will put you in the exercise category that is going to do the most good to increase your heart to build its strength. Since everyone has a different starting point in age and conditioning, it is necessary to make correct calculations for each individual. (Cathy Smith, WalkFit for a Better Body, P 33)

Target Training Zones

Target Training Zones	
Age	Target Zone
20	120 - 160
25	117 - 156
30	114 - 152
35	111 - 148
40	108 - 144
45	105 - 140
50	102 - 136
55	99 - 132
60	96 - 124
65	93 - 124
70	90 - 120
75+	87 - 116

Again, I find this chart, from Cathy Smith's Walkfit for a Better Body, very helpful and it takes away the mystery of it all. The idea is to start where you are and build the strength of that heart. If you have any existing heart condition you should be under the guidance of your health care professional, so that you gain heart strength, rather than hurting yourself.

For example if you are age 40, your maximum heart rate is approximately 180. Take 60% of 180 (108) for the low end, and 80% (which is 144) for the high end. Then try to walk at a pace that keeps your heart rate above 108, but below 144. This will put you in the exercise category that is going to do the most good to increase your heart to build its strength. Since everyone has a different starting point in age and conditioning, it is necessary to make correct calculations for each individual. (Cathy Smith, WalkFit for a Better Body, P 33)

8 to 10 hours of sleep/ 24 hrs or at least bed rest are essential if you want your heart to remain healthy. Stress cannot be eliminated, but rest is a time of rebuilding. Learn what causes your stress. Look for ways to prevent it. Sometimes it is a matter of mental attitude, such as The Little Engine That Could. The little train in the story always believed he could do whatever he had to do.

Our present day stresses are often a result of a feeling of incompetence—or that we will not be able to do what we are called upon to do. Impatience with one's self sets in and is often transferred to others such as happens in the epidemic of "road rage" happening all across American highways. Don't ignore the important factor of purposeful stress reduction for heart health.

Life Expectancy
Yet if you " Adopt Dr. Willix's way of looking at health, . . . there is no biological reason why you can't live to be over 100." (Maximum Health, Robert D. Willix, Jr, M.D. Introduction) In addition to changing your heart diet and heart lifestyle, there is one more aspect that needs to be considered. It involves the concept of not eating so much. (Denham Harman- Free Radical Theory)

Here in America where heart disease is the highest in the world, we have an abundance of food and as great a lack of self discipline. Exposure to TV promotions is a problem. "The incidence of . . . vascular disease and heart disease respectively is 63% and 96% in normally fed rats, but only . . . 10% and 26% in diet restricted rats. A high incidence of arteriosclerosis occurs normally in certain strains of pigeons, but can be greatly diminished by under nutrition."

In animals there are a number of bio-markers that determine biological age as opposed to chronological age. These include cholesterol increase, contractibility of heated collagen (the main chemical component of connective tissue) and liver enzymes. Dr Walford, MD sets the expected age of those with restricted caloric diets, to be an easy 120 years, barring accidents.

The immune system:
This system declines with age due to the fact that the body does not differentiate the "self" and "non-self" cells as readily, and as a result, can begin to self destruct through antibodies and lymphocytes. It is this distinction that is not clear as one ages, so that you have a reduced ability in the immune response as well as a reduced ability to repair damaged or faulty cells. These two processes are greatly improved by a simple reduction in the total caloric intake, yet maintaining a high nutritional content.

To understand more of this concept I would recommend Dr. Walford's research, for it has been established that under-nutrition proves quite the opposite of mal-nutrition. The brain continues to develop and all body functions are enhanced when the diet consists of less calories but more nutritious value. I have often said while shopping for organic foods, "I guess we will just have to eat less, but keep the value high." (Max Life Span, R.L. Walford, 104-10)

This section is typical of a Nutrition course for students intending this as a career.

Obviously the optometrist will be interested in it both from a personal aspect for the help it might provide in managing one's own health, but will wish his patients and registrants to benefit from much of the knowledge it contains.

Realistically that would be an unattainable ideal. We have too many procedures and notes to make to indulge ourselves in educating everyone. Nor do all wish to be burdened with extra knowledge, especially if it is not seen as immediately relevant for the purpose of CardioRetinometry®.

Many take the view that "ignorance is bliss" and want it to remain so. One must have a solid grid or foundation on which to build health. Otherwise we have a system of band aids to cover up or alleviate symptoms in the short term. In other words supplements in large doses can also be used pharmaceutically, to bring immediate results that will not endure.

We are looking for the long haul as Dr Bush demonstrates for those who will be consistent. One needs to follow through for many years in order to prevent life threatening events from shortening the life or bringing about a poor quality of life. He and his registrants have proven what works.

With that in mind the below is offered more to complete the essentials of a course in nutrition, with significant value for examination purposes for the planned Doctorate in CardioRetinometry® degree.

Four Friendly Doctors

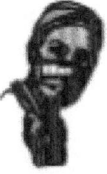 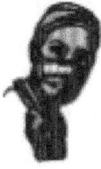 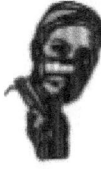 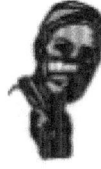

Dr	Dr	Dr	Dr
Cleanse	Oxygen	Nourish	Balance

A deficiency or disease, anywhere or of any type, in or on the body, is a sign that the tissues have not received enough oxygen and that the immune system has been overtaxed. It has become ineffective in destroying unhealthy cells or invading pathogens, bacteria, viruses, and fungi, as well as malfunction of one or more major glands in the endocrine system, necessary for sustenance of an efficiently operating body.

Cancer

There are perhaps 200 different causes of cancer.
These cells have been changed in their ability to replicate healthy cells and therefore thrive on carbon dioxide, a waste product of the human body. This knowledge was discovered by Otto Warburg in the 1930's, which earned him the Nobel Prize for finding one answer to the puzzle of the cause of cancer. From Warburg's discovery we know that cancer cells ferment sugar.

This valuable information can mean the difference between life and death; a pain-ridden - or - a pain free zest for life versus hopelessness.

It is from this basis that I present some ways by

which we can take charge of our own lives and use the God given ability which we all posses - to do something about our own health and that of our families. A general guideline to remember when one has been diagnosed as having any condition that is all the way from "just uncomfortable" to a life threatening disease. We have four doctors who will help our bodies heal.

I'll introduce you to each of them in turn.
If I had any of the diet related diseases listed at the beginning of this book, I would go to all four of these wonderful healing Doctors, because they help the body heal itself.

Dr. Cleanse
He is a very knowledgeable doctor regarding healing the body. You take charge yourself. Cleanse the body of toxins, chemicals, pathogens, bacteria, viruses, mucous, phlegm, parasites, etc. When tissues are healthy with adequate ascorbate, they can throw off many toxins. One theory seeks to nourish the body to produce healthy cells - a second theory states that if the cells are clean, they will healthily fight off disease.
It might be in your best interest to work with your Health Care Professional who is trained and well versed in the cleansing processes as outlined in Dr. Bernard Jensen' book *Tissue Cleansing Through Bowel Management*. Think of it this way. If you did not like the putrid exhaust coming out of your automobile's exhaust pipe, you would not go back there and try to clean up that exhaust. No. You would stop the engine and have it checked out to find the cause of the toxic emission and correct it from inside the engine. It is no different with your body. Any illness calls for a thorough cleansing of all cells, and organs of elimination.

Laxative:

Begin with a good herbal laxative to cleanse the lower colon. There are several on the market, but it should include Cascara Sagrada as a main ingredient. Take this the night before you begin your cleansing program, and you will have a good start. These herbs are not chemically laxative so that long term use doesn't create dependency, as can happen with chemical purgatives.

The following chart will work in conjunction with either a daily cleansing with a colema board, or you can use high enemas that will reach little by little up into the entire large intestine. This is done without any ballooning or pressure and the water is expelled as soon as the urge is felt, to prevent discomfort. If you get a colema board, the full directions come with it.

Colema:

A colema board will put you in charge of your own "cleansing clinic"so to speak. If you cannot obtain one of these you can use a high enema although it is neither as easy nor effective as the colema, it is better than nothing. Colema boards are made by several companies. One is the Ultimate Colonic Unit, by Ultimate Trends, Inc, 7835 South 1300 East, Sandy, Utah 84094, 1-800-745-3191 as advertised in Let's Live, June 1992.

A High Enema is composed of as many as five enema bags being taken into the bowel, one after the other and expelled when needed. When the water is in the bowel, the person takes the knee-chest position and massages the lower abdomen from the left lower side, up across the transverse colon and down to the area on the right side where the appendix or ileocecal valve is.

This exercise loosens all impacted putrid material so that it can be expelled. If there is soreness in the bowel, one can add a cup of Alfa-Mint tea to sooth the bowel walls; one quarter cup of the mucilage from soaked flax seeds for soothing; or one quarter cup Bentonite clay water which assists in soaking up toxins and then getting them out of the colon.

There are products which, when taken orally, will help dissolve any sticky, compacted residue in the bowel walls. One such is called Homozon. Aloe Vera may also be useful for this purpose.

This is a seven Day Program. The first day is different from the second day and the next five are all the same and will be given in that order. It is taken from the ideas given by Dr. Bernard Jensen. An easy chart designed by Fanie Carriere of Indianola, WA, has been a real help to those who pursue this cleansing program. (Erickson,Ten Major Causes of Death and Disease ..., Pp 55,56....)

You need to prepare the Flaxseed the night before. Soak ½ cup Flaxseed in a one quart jar filled with hot, pure warm water. Let it soak 8 hours for use the next day. Then strain it and use only the mucilage. You can discard the seeds. Cold soak Oats the night before use.

Dr. Oxygen
This doctor gives you the most important nutrient you need to keep living. Only four minutes without it and your brain cells begin to die.

It would be so life giving to you if you could begin to grow wheat grass, harvest it, and make juice from it. It is a powerful healing modality in cases of cancer as proven by the Hippocrates Institute in Florida, (administrator, Ann Wigmore).

Get a planting tray with a clear cover for it. Fill it with good potting soil, organically composted if possible. Sprinkle over the top of the soil a layer of Red Wheat kernels. Press them down but not under the soil. Water well. Cover with a clear lid and cover with a dark towel. Let it germinate and grow to seven inches high, when it is ready to harvest.

You can get a mechanical or electric juicer that extracts the juice by pressure rather than centrifugal force - much more juice is obtained than in a regular juicer. Drink two ounces of this juice in the morning and two ounces in the evening. It is powerful and health giving because it is full of chlorophyll, besides being alive.

Sprouting
Get a booklet on sprouting at your health store. It will tell you exactly how to sprout all kinds of seeds. These seeds have the gift of life in them, because in the sprouting process they are alive and growing. They are life giving. Eat as many as you like. You can use them in salads, sandwiches, alone, or on cereals, etc. You can also put them in the blender, in vegetable juice, soy, nut, oat or rice "milk" drinks.

Oxygen/Ozone
To get oxygen to the cells of the body is vastly important because no cancer cell can live in the presence of oxygen. As mentioned, in 1931 a Nobel

Prize was given to Otto Warburg, the scientist who discovered a cause of cancer, i.e., the lack of oxygen causing anaerobic glycolysis. That is one of the reasons why smoking is so debilitating to one's health; because it cuts off the oxygen we depend on for everything. Free radicals then provide the energy the cells need for the glycolysis, but antioxidants quenching the free radicals prevent this and the cancer then dies.

Second hand smoke is even worse for our health, because we are breathing unfiltered smoke directly from the burning end of the cigarette It is so vital to full recovery that I am sad when some can't buy the *Æthozol System*, which provides this drastically important 'nutrient.' We can only live four minutes without oxygen before the brain begins to die, whereas we can live much longer without food or water. In the form of O_3 (ozone) it can be taken by colonic infusion, 250 cc daily for 30 consecutive days and then repeated after resting for a week. Warning; No smoking when working with oxygen!

Cancer

The following more detailed explanation is taken from Dr. Bush's encyclopaedia, "700 Vitamin C Secrets." and is used by permission.
"Cancer, growth:
Accelerated by intermediate doses of vitamin C, e.g. 5 grams/day before being retarded and stopped by higher doses. I am grateful to Dr David W. Gregg PhD for his hypothesis, stimulated by the work of Dr. Arthur B. Robinson MD which I feel is worthy of study. His paper is found on www.nutritionandcancer.org

"Dr. Robinson reports that vitamin C in ordinary doses accelerated the growth of cancer. This is consistent with other reports where it was found that tumours do consume vitamin C from blood. These two pieces of information would indicate that cancer cells have a way of metabolizing vitamin C, enhancing growth. The evidence was convincing to me and I decided to see if I could identify the biochemical mechanism. Instead of invoking an unknown mechanism I thought I would start by considering the biochemical sequence that produces collagen, which is known to require vitamin C. This sequence requires both vitamin C and alpha ketoglutarate. Alpha ketoglutarate is produced by the fourth step of the citric acid cycle along with the first molecule of NADH. The vitamin C alpha ketoglutarate and the molecule of NADH are required for the side chain that produces collagen. However, the rest of the citric acid cycle is blocked at this point. Further steps produce more NADH and FADH2 both of which can be utilized only in the following respiratory chain. That is where, in aerobic metabolism, oxygen is reacted with the hydrogen on NADH and FADH2 to make water, producing enough energy to provide 33 of the 36 (adenosine) ATPs.

Since, for the anaerobic cancer cells, oxygen transport to the cells is blocked, the respiratory chain is also blocked. A blockage of the citric acid cycle here causes build-up of alpha ketoglutarate. This build-up will stimulate the side reaction producing collagen, requiring and consuming vitamin C. This side reaction also allows more of the earlier, anaerobic glycolysis to take place which provides two ATPs of energy per glucose molecule consumed. The combination of producing collagen, a vital cellular building block, and a quite modest amount of additional energy could promote the growth of cancer. Thus, one could explain how modest doses of vitamin C could promote the growth of cancer."

Also see. http://www.krysalis.net/cancer4.htm Dr Robinson's article on 'krysalis' I would emphasise that

Dr. Robinson states, that "Vitamin C at ordinary doses (human equivalents of 1 to 5 grams/day) increased the growth rate of cancer while far larger doses suppressed the cancer growth rate."

Sydney Bush's note:
"I have never taken less than 20 grams/day of sodium L-ascorbate for the last 20 years. The body draws what it wants from the gut. The rest was 'geographically' in the body but not in the physiological sense until it passes out of the gut into the blood stream. This is one of the many reasons why I have always urged people to never use tablets as their main source but to use the bulk powder. Thank you Dr. Robinson."

Respiration
In the form of O_3 (*Æthozol*), it can be taken by respiratory inhalation for 20 to 30 minutes per day. Directions must be followed specifically as per health care practitioner's instructions. (C10 H10 03)

Insufflation
Insufflations can be continued for 30 days and suspended for one week as stated above. Then this

Cycle can be resumed and repeated for three months. After that it can be reduced to once every other day for continued maintenance, until the immune system is rebuilt through good nutrition and food supplementation. This usually takes three months to turn around. The changed diet must become a way of life because the old way was producing deficiencies and made the body susceptible to degenerated or faulty cells.

Flooding our bodies with oxygen is going to be a continuing way of life. The body renews some cells in a short time. Others don't replicate for 5 or 10 years. We want to continue on a good health program for life so that all faulty cells are replaced with good ones. Then we will not be hosts to bacteria, fungus types, viruses and pathogens.

The Æthozol System:
The fastest surest way is to use the *Æthozol System* which gives 250 cc of ozone (made from pure oxygen) per insufflation. It can be self administered into the colon where it goes directly into the blood stream via the portal vein, and thence to the liver. Respiration will deliver ozone in the form of Æthozol O_8, to the pulmonary veins in the lungs. An Oitic device allows for insufflation to the ear, and will get oxygen into the blood from the tiny network of blood vessels there. (William A. Turska, NMD, *Æthozol Technical Manual*, Scandia Publishers, Silverdale, WA, 1993, pages 5-8)
Some Alternative care Physicians give ozone treatments by withdrawing blood, ozonating it and re-injecting it back into the patient. This is usually done in a series which is determined by the doctor and the condition for which one is being treated. It is widely used in Germany for cancer, AIDS, and stroke

recovery among many other conditions. One should consult a qualified health care professional to administer this treatment in conjunction with dietary and other means of returning to health. Ozone Therapy is now legal in several states where it cannot be denied to those who wish it.

Water with Food Grade H_2O_2

The following directions were given to me by the late Dr William Turska, NMD. For one gallon of distilled water add 144 drops of 35% food grade Hydrogen peroxide (H_2O_2) to make a 3% solution.

Food grade does not contain preservatives as the 3 % found in retail stores. H_2O_2 (35% food grade) can be obtained from chemical companies and is now available in some health store outlets.

It can be taken in water in carefully measured drops. Begin with 9 drops per 8 ounce glass of purified water. If this is tolerated without nausea, then increase it by a drop per day until reaching the limit of tolerance. i.e., no nausea. A therapeutic dose would be 25 drops per 8 ounce glass - taken three times per day. Depending on one's size and weight, tolerance varies with the individual.

This product causes a bubbly sensation in the mouth, hence the feeling of nausea. Do not try to exceed your limit. The dosage is for a therapy i.e., if one has a serious health condition.

For daily maintenance or for purifying drinking water it is not necessary to use 35%. You can safely use 3% and shouldn't experience nausea or use ascorbic acid.

For those who cannot tolerate oxygen in this form there is stabilized oxygen as a supplement, and *Homozon* or *San-O-Zone,* which create nascent oxygen to be ingested or for bathing. Both are mixed with lemon juice which activates the powder and releases newly formed, life giving oxygen. These were used by Dr. Blass years ago and are still available from the International Association of Oxygen Therapy, a division of American Society of Medical Missionaries, P.O. Box 1360, Priest River, ID 83856.

H_2O_2 Intravenous injections:

This product goes into the blood stream and can benefit all areas of the body where cancer or other debilitating problems may be. This must be administered by a qualified health care professional.

H_2O_2 Other products:

In any illness, or for prevention, the main objective is to get oxygen to the cells in as many ways as possible. This can also be done by taking green *Spirulina*, eating raw vegetables, sprouted seed and grains, especially dark green "veggies" for chlorophyll and yellow ones for beta carotene. All are mentioned separately above. Of course, wheat grass juice and all sprouted seeds will deliver oxygen to the cells, so be sure to include them in your daily diet.

It is easy to sprout seeds in your own kitchen, so you can have fresh foods every day without worrying about them spoiling before you eat them, such as is the case with so many vegetables we have to buy by the "head" or "stalk."

Oxygen

Dr. Kurt Donsbach has published a book, *Oxygen,*

Oxygen, Oxygen which gives various applications of oxygen/ozone therapies. Ed Mc.Cabe has published a book, *Oxygen Therapies.* Both are helpful in understanding more about the subject. There is a vast amount of literature available about this wonderful health helper. Elizabeth Baker writes *The Un-Medical Miracle-Oxygen,* which is also excellent.

The Second Opinion Doctor, William Campbell Douglas, MD has written *Hydrogen Peroxide Medical Miracle* where he also tells about Luminescent Therapy using ultra violet light to cleanse the blood. It is excellent reading, as well as "hope giving."

Dr. Nourish

This doctor will take you on your way to a life full of vigor, and vitality for a high quality long life.

Soy Products.
Soy has been used extensively for centuries. Orientals used it long before it came into use in the Western world. However the Japanese used it as a fermented food and used it very sparingly with perhaps 1 to 2 teaspoons per day, compared to the western world now having laced soy into every imaginable product especially processed foods, making the daily intake far beyond what other nations have ever used per day.

Tofu
They have used Tofu, a soy product, in all kinds of drinks, soups, salads, etc. It is a reasonably healthy food and was to provide protein, when not eating red meat. Some in the west have substituted soy for red meat which has left vegetarians without the needed nutrients to keep a balanced nutritional program.

While filling their children with much too high estrogenic factors in their diet they have traded for these adverse effects, such as the sexual development, disrupted monthly cycles for women and infertility as well as promoting cancers and many other adverse health conditions.

The Meat Mistake
This was done inadvertently to avoid the meat consumption of animals fed and raised on synthetic hormones, herbicides and inorganic, fertilized feed. Soya beans are not immune to this of course. Many of the crops are now genetically engineered, full of overspray from herbicides and unfit for human consumption.

Soy that is acceptable is fermented and includes Natto containing Vitamin K for blood clotting and building strong bones. Tempo, Miso and Soy Sauce if produced properly, are healthful additions to one's diet when used in moderation as the Orientals have done for centuries.

Goitrogens
In addition according to Dr Mercola's report, soy contains aluminium, hemaglutinin which promotes clots and clumping of blood cells and goitrogens harming the thyroid, as well as phytates which prevent mineral absorption and is also loaded with genistein and daidzein blocking estrogen on the other hand.

Daily intake should be no more than 30 grams per day and that should be in the form of fermented soy for best health results. Vitamin C may help a little.

Early puberty

Soy has estrogenic factors and can bring about early puberty in children and should not be used as a replacement for milk. Some nutritionists believe that this also causes excess estrogen in young people resulting in questions or confusion about their gender.

The New Zealand government put warnings on soy milk cartons not to give to children due to premature puberty. One rule for unknown factors is "when in doubt, don't." Just as with so many warnings for health safety, use your own reasoning and be safe. Our food and water sources are so polluted that it pays to be careful. For example, when water is left in plastic bottles, especially in a vehicle trunk where it gets heated, it can cause many adverse biological reactions that cause early puberty. Cooking in Microwave ovens with plastic is another questionable practice, further increasing the estrogen we ingest.

Cell Phones

Another example of safety is the use of cell phones which in very many studies have proven detrimental to the brain. The other warning ignored by many is the use of tobacco products. Many years later the damage has often reached the point of no return. My personal thought is, if the jury is still out, then don't follow the questionable practice. No risk in health concerns should be dismissed lightly for a few minutes of pleasure or convenience. Years later your body will make you answer for everything you put into it.

Additional information on the use of Vitamin C:
Vitamin C has been shown to be vital in treating many conditions. Essential for phagocytosis and radiation protection, Klenner stated that it kills all viruses!

Vitamin C (Sodium Ascorbate)

20 grams per day (20,000 milligrams) can be tolerated by many people in divided doses. Some need much less, the frequency being more important for everyone who needs it. Some people need it twice daily and others every hour or two especially with aging. Changes in the bowel habit help to determine what type of person you are, but the only certain way is to either test the urine several times per day, or seek CardioRetinometry® for the complete picture. What matters most is how one's arteries are clogging! One might measure one's vitamin C but a good result does not have to last much more than three or four hours. So it can be misleading unless it is measured perhaps, four times per day.

Vitamin C in each 24 hour period.

Good advice is to dissolve it in water and then one can sip it all day and into the evening. It can also be drunk quickly with juice or water. The 'neutralized' sodium ascorbate form is preferred as the ascorbic acid form, like fruit juices, can attack the dentine of the teeth.

How to Increase dietary Vitamin C

One example for many with sensitive reactions to laxative foods is that a flat teaspoon of Vitamin C is usually 2 to 2.2 grams (2,000 to 2,200mgs) and should be taken at the rate of 1/4 tsp per day for 4 or 5 days, increasing to ½ tsp for 3 - 4 more days. Animals have the huge advantage over us of injecting themselves continuously with it from the liver. We cannot do that. Stress the goat and its production will leap from half a gram per hour to four grams per hour automatically. We can beat rate limited goats by taking pure powder to reach bowel intolerance again.

One can find – depending on one's age – that where a gram five times per day might loosen the bowels generally, and certainly a gram or two or three in the early morning can have the desired effect, this bowel response can be lost during stress.

It has been reported that for unknown reasons a normal 5 grams/day bowel tolerance limit can suddenly require ten grams every hour for a day before reaching bowel intolerance again!

What illness was pre-empted?

At exceptional times like this one might take as much as 100 or even 200 grams before a bowel action is restored. What does it mean? We can only guess that some toxin, bacterium or virus was absorbing all the vitamin C. Dr. Hugh Riordan, being tested daily and bitten by a spider became anascorbemic, losing ALL his blood vitamin C for five days. At the time he was being closely monitored every day for other research. He was immediately administered 12 grams per day by injection before it became measurable in his blood stream again on the fifth day. Why they didn't inject more as Dr. Klenner would have done, we don't know.

Gradual increase.

Increase to 3/4 tsp for 3 - 4 more days
Increase to level teaspoon for 3 - 4 days
Increase to rounded teaspoon

From here one can continue to increase the amount up to 20 grams or more per day, which would be 5 rounded teaspoons per day. The key to one's personal tolerance level, is, as we all learn, the bowel effect. In the progression, if diarrhea occurs, then decrease to the previous level until abated. No lasting damage can occur.

If diarrhea has occurred you need to increase the trace minerals, especially potassium, and drink plenty of water. It might be wise to take 99 mg to 400 mg of Potassium for a day or two, to replace that most important mineral so as to avoid any possible muscles cramps due to its loss when losing large amounts of water from the body. If you can tolerate bananas they are high in potassium as is orange juice. The Atkins diet which is diuretic recommends even more potassium.

New Knowledge about vitamin C.
The following is taken from Dr. Bush's encyclopaedia. As yet the erythroidal re-reduction of oxidised vitamin C discovered by Montel-Hagen, Sitbon and Taylor, appears, for reasons we can't understand, to be unreported elsewhere with the expected great fanfare of publicity.

Dynamic flow model:
Building on the work of Klenner, Cathcart, Pauling, Stone, Fonorow and others, Hickey and Roberts take the thinking further and suggest, very reasonably, one must agree, that the dynamic flow model makes sense of many of the clinical observations of the effects of ascorbate over the whole range of intakes of vitamin C. We naturally seek to demonstrate that the results of experiment are consistent with the model. In an extensive search of the literature they failed to discover any experimental or clinical studies that do not comply with its predictions. Working towards a better understanding of antioxidant function, they state that Dynamic Flow restores human physiology to the condition of animals that synthesise their own vitamin C. Unfortunately, the work of May, Qu and

Whitesell of 1995 followed by the aforementioned startling discovery of Montel-Hagen, Sitbon and Taylor published this month, April 2009 (the encyclopedia was published in October 2010) may compel us to modify that view. It now appears that, at least below renal threshold (for it is a biphasic system and this is now what I am sure others must join me in suggesting for a reasonable modus operandi, because we agree that we see the continuous excretion of ascorbate as essential for a healthy urogenital system when we have spare) the blood can now be seen to be acting as a unitary organ maintaining a constant optimised ratio of ascorbate to dehydroascorbate for its continued desirable vitamin C excretion.

As Montel-Hagen, Sitbon and Taylor say in this most recent discovery not yet reported in the media although now nearly a month old, "it had always been assumed" that mammalian blood of all species behaved in the same way. But, as they point out, they found a 'dramatic' difference in that only in human's does erythroidal glutathione recycling of the monodehydroascorbate anion take place in the red cell's cytoplasm with return to the plasma of L-ascorbic acid. To add to the complexity of the dynamic flow model, May, Qu and Whitesell (a haematologist doctor with a sense of humour) found that, acting as a unitary organ, the erythroidal component of whole blood is able to re-reduce the entire monodehydro-ascorbate anion of the system for conserving vitamin C and to reprocess the entire plasma complement every three minutes. In addition it appears that there are further differences which require investigation. Of course this means that, rather than being disadvantaged compared with the animals and, given the intelligence to use vitamin C optimally to provide a constant 1,000 times more than we need in our gut as a reservoir, it seems that we can meet and overcome challenges that would kill the animals that are rate limited in their production. Indeed, the reason why not all are killed by new strains of infections for which nobody possesses antibodies, may be that a limited number of extremely blessed individuals, enjoying the best of both worlds, can make extra vitamin C whilst drawing on that provided by a sensible diet chosen for a rainy day. The popular saying "Everything in moderation," is then seen as suicidal, showing little understanding of the facts or a sentence of death for a child if it is the dictum of doctors or parents. Klenner would have none of that. May J.M, Qu Z.C, Whitesell R.R. *Ascorbic acid recycling enhances the antioxidant reserve of human erythrocytes.* Biochemistry. 1995 Oct 3;34(39):12721-8. See dynamic flow.

Enzymes
After age 25, enzymes are limited in the body due to the habit of eating cooked foods. We must replace them through supplements. If one is already well and just wanting to have a little assistance with digestion there are many others on the market. My choice would include the necessary enzymes to digest all vegetable, grain and fruit fibers - lipase, protease, and cellulase as well as pancreatin and ox bile for the digestion of meats and proteins.

Total digestion means that one has more energy because there is less gastric disturbance, better assimilation and less stress on other body systems, for example the heart, liver, and the pancreas. If you are not able to get this product from your health care professional, then you could get Betaine Hydrochloride from a health store, or natural health department of a pharmacy or grocery.

Betaine Hydrochloride with Pepsin.

This is an excellent digestion and assimilation aid and assists the body, which may be lacking in hydrochloric acid. It declines in everyone from about age 25 and should be taken with each meal. In addition enzymes from Papaya and Bromelain, (papaya and pineapple enzymes), may be taken with each meal.

Acid Indegestion

Amazingly, when we have what we interpret as "acid indigestion" it is most often caused by *too little* stomach acid to digest the food. Then you have an eruption of gases from partially digested foods. Yes; the antacids *calm the storm*, but do not address the origin of the problem which is almost a definition of allopathic medicine, addressing symptoms more than causes.

Vitamin E

This is a known anti-oxidant in cancer prevention or treatment. See the five different types of Vitamin E listed earlier in this document. There are only 2 on the market that can be taken in large enough quantities to do the job. These are *Unique E* (from Grace Co in Texas) and *A&E Mulsins* (from Germany). *Unique E,* take 2400 mg per day all at once in the morning with a glass of water.

.

Warning: Do not take any other Vitamin E at this high dose because it can cause serious problems due to the possibility of rancid oils in the capsules. Other E supplements can also cause problems with rise in blood pressure unless gradually building up to about 800 to 1,000 IU per day. It may not be easy to find but I advise a capsule formulated with glycerol is better than soy oil. It must be natural and say d-alpha tocopherol on the label. I repeat because it is so very important - Dl-alpha tocopherol (or dl-alpha tocopherol) is synthetic and a waste of health and money. Too often it is used in $Million studies and now we don't need to spend time wondering why? It is so easy to design studies on nutrition to produce any desired result. It is not unknown for pharmacists, to profess that they knew no difference.

Oatmeal (raw or warmed to not over 150 º F)

Take one serving per day, especially in winter. The reasons are multitudinous, but mainly oatmeal is an antibacterial, anti fungal and anti virus food. It builds and maintains energy. It helps provide the needed bulk for good bowel health. To prepare a strength giving drink, take ½ cup raw, non-instant Oatmeal. Soak overnight in 1 quart of purified or distilled water. In the morning, strain off and drink that liquid throughout the day. It will give endurance and energy. It was used in times past for threshing crews, between meals to help them work until the noon or evening meal was served.

Acidophilus

Acidophilus can be taken as tablets or liquid. One needs to build this up so that food can be properly assimilated as well as being digested. After building up the bowel climate to the correct friendly bacteria (acidophilus) it can be maintained by taking unsweetened, non-fruit yogurt. For those intolerant to lactose acidophilus can be obtained from strawberries.

Make sure the label says the acidophilus is active or live. It is necessary to maintain a good climate in the bowel for maximum health. Everyone used to know that, but for the last 50 yrs and Freud's teaching equated bowel movements with sexual gratification, there has been shame connected to this important organ and people have avoided discussion on bowel regularity. The faulty teaching has been disseminated from many health care professionals that one bowel movement every few days is okay. It is not okay! The entire animal kingdom evacuates after each meal, while we humans think it is healthy to have as many as 9 meals backed up in the colon before we admit something is wrong. Then most use chemical laxatives to correct something that needs correcting from the diet and lifestyle. Read *Tissue Cleansing Through Bowel Management* by Dr. Jensen. You will be shocked--and convinced about the need for bowel management, if you plan to be healthy and long lived.

Flax Seed Oil
Take at least one tablespoon small curd (avoid large curd) cottage cheese, once per day with 1 teaspoon of *Flax Seed Oil* mixed in. It is quite pleasant. The cottage cheese is a high sulpha food. Together they have also been used in cancer treatments for many years, by Nobel prize nominee Joanna Budwig, and also nourishes the skin, prostate and other organ systems in the body.

Food Changes
Eat and drink all the green foods you can for chlorophyll, and phytonutrients. *Spirulina Plankton* mixed in a little juice is excellent. I like to use 2 ounces of almond. rice milk, or apple juice to mix the *Spirulina* in and drink it down with a "chaser" of plain juice. There are a number of other sources of

chlorophyll, e.g., wheat grass juice, barley green, blue green algae, alfalfa and all green vegetables, especially the darkest green ones. Wheat grass juice has been used in the Hippocrates Institute for many years. It gets the fresh growing plant essence directly to the cells most effectively. Some *juice bars* grow and process this life giving juice on a daily basis. Otherwise you can grow and juice your own, but you need a special juicer to extract the juice. Some who could not get a juicer have used their blender and drank the whole wheat grass, pulp and all.

Nebuchadnezzar in the Old Testament, when mentally ill, ate grass in the field, like an ox. Later He was delivered from his mental disease. There have been other testimonies of people eating the grass itself and experiencing better health and quicker healing from accidents.

Raw carrot juice
Mixed with Beet and Cucumber juice are also excellent health builders and cleansers. Celery juice is also a tremendous cell cleanser. You will feel fresh and clean inside when you drink these life giving juices.

Raw foods provide the extra needed enzymes to digest them as well as better absorption, and getting extra oxygen to the cells. Live foods are the important issue to regain or maintain good health, preventing many ills and much pain. We must partake of the best foods we can get.

If one is very ill, in seeking to enhance any area of health, one may have to eliminate all meats for a time, adding back only fish and chicken - - and that only three times per week.

Here's a note to tuck away in your "thinking cap" for future reference: *Proteins must be obtained from a vegetarian like diet while fighting such a debilitating diseases as cancer and other serious disorders.*

Sugars

Refined beet and cane sugars <u>must be eliminated</u> as well as white flour and all processed foods. Sugar content should be less than 12 grams; 7 or 8 are even better. Fat intake should be cut back to no more than 2 grams or 20% per serving. High triglycerides are caused by too much sugar or simple carbohydrates. It is these foods that cause plaque build up rather than fats, if you are consuming healthy fats, e.g., butter instead of margarine; olive, flax or coconut oil instead of corn or soy, etc..

Make a "label reading trip" around your grocery store. Patients with "type O" blood can tolerate more fat but no blood type can tolerate sugar. It is a drug and should be avoided except for unheated, unrefined honey and that in moderation. Even sugars in fruits must be monitored by diabetics who are watching their blood glucose.

Drinks

Coffee, and other drinks containing caffeine, chocolate, and black tea should be avoided. A new study was presented on Dr Mercola's e-Newsletter praising coffee for many health benefits, but remember the jury is still out on that. Do not jump on every bandwagon that comes along for natural health. The exception of course is herb teas which have healing properties, researched for generations, in many countries world wide. Green tea may be taken if you pour the boiling water over the bag or leaves, let stand one minute, pour off and immerse tea in a new cup of water to steep before drinking. This will "decaffeinate" the tea as the Orientals do.

Of course, in any return to health, all alcoholic beverages must be eliminated. If you could see what contortions the liver must go through to eliminate alcoholic beverages from your body, you would never put another drop in your body. (Ref. a study by the Psychology Department at University of Colorado Boulder) Let's vote for the liver today, since it has more than 500 jobs to do already, and "give it a break!"

Oxygen:
Remember we can live for many days without food, we can live for a number of days without water, but to deprive us of oxygen for four minutes will result in brain damage that is often irreversible. So, in a way, oxygen is our most important nutrient!

Pantothenic Acid 100 mg per day
If you are taking a multiple vitamin mineral, make sure you are taking the correct amount. You should be getting 100 mg daily of this important vitamin. It has been found to be effective, acting, like vitamin C as a natural antihistamine. It has also been used successfully in dealing with auto-immune responses, such as arthritis, post nasal drip, shortness of breath, nasal obstructions and cysts, and is an important factor in hair growth., etc.

CoQ10 (Coenzyme Q 10) 60 to 100 mg daily
This is a proven enhancement to all body functions and has been used in anti-cancer diets.

Its importance increases significantly with age as it involves the 'heartbeat' and levels may have been inhibited by statin medications before registrants learned of their dangers. We cannot countermand medically prescribed drugs and must avoid friction with our medical colleagues. Patients can ask their doctors to help them wean off these strong drugs.

Herbs:

There has been great success in promoting healing and health through the use of herbs for many centuries. The following are some of the best. All are not available in all areas, hence the listing of several kinds. If you have believed that we live longer now, check out the ages of most of our early legislators. Many lived into the 80's and 90's. They had good food.

Many who went west in settling America, did not have good food and we have come to believe on the basis of their early deaths, that ours must be short also. Many people who reach 60 think they will die by 70 so they program their bodies to do just that. With herbal remedies and supplementation there is no need for an early death, or compromised quality of life.

Creosote Bush tea (Chaparral) *has been used in successful cancer treatments.*
at the Brigham Young University in Utah.
Ginseng 2000 mg per day, tea, capsules or extract. There are six kinds of ginsengs so don't short yourself by only taking one kind.
American
Chinese
Japanese
Korean

Siberian
Teinchi
Pau d'Arco tea 4 cups per day, used successfully in cancer treatments, and is a great detoxifier.
Red Clover tea or capsules or extract
Burdock Root teas, capsules or extract
Yellow Dock Root tea, capsules or extract
waters, enema waters, poultices, hot packs called fomentations, to breathe in steam, topical applications, etc. If you want to study herbs seriously, there are many other books available including Culpepper's herbal works.

Herbs for Depression:
Sometimes stress results in low level depression that we don't often recognize. If depressed, drink *Licorice* root tea, Astragalus. It is important to work with the body so that it can heal itself. Other herbs for depression are *Kava Kava* and *St John's Wort* (Hypericum). St Johns' Wort also is useful in bladder control. Used in conjunction with Yarrow and Pipsissewa you will have your leakage problem under control again. The first and most important thing to think about in any recovery program, after adequate vitamin C (scurvy causing apathy) is to cleanse the 5 major eliminative organs. These are

1. Lungs,
2. Skin,
3. Liver
4. Kidneys,
5. Bowels

Dr. Balance
For ongoing health, Dr. Balance will work with you as you learn to "listen to your body."

It is a matter of fine tuning an efficient machine.
Indeed, you are an electrical, mechanical, biochemical, spiritual being.
Things don't just happen, they are caused. Now the fun begins. You are well on your way to the best.
Blue Violet extract
Golden Seal Root - use the whole plant for Pancreas

Immune System
Echinacea tea, capsules or extract (an immune system enhancer)
Aloes
Comfrey tea or capsules
Blue Flag tea or capsules
Dandelion Root (especially good for the Pancreas)

Heart health and Cayenne
African Cayenne, a wonderful healing herb is not really in the pepper family. Good for the Pancreas as well as a heart regulator and astringent.

Healing
Chickweed tea or capsules - another wonderful healing herb
That is extra good for weight loss and a diuretic.
Rock Rose
Oregon Grape tea or capsules
Agrimony
Blueberry Leaves tea or capsules,

A Great Astringent
Blueberry Roots are nature's strongest astringent to stop bleeding.
Huckleberry Leaves tea or capsules

Sources of Herbal Information

Excellent instruction on the use of herbs can be found in *Back to Eden* by Jethro Kloss. *The Complete Medicinal Herbal* by Penelope Ody is excellent as it gives the part of the herb to be used as well as the time to harvest and the way to prepare for various applications and uses. Herbal teas can be added to the bath and are available World-wide (Managed Health Care)

<u>You</u> are the Manager!!

Everyone has something to manage and the excellence of that management determines how well one feels, and how easily the required tasks for each day are executed. Don't ever let anyone put you down, or assume that you don't feel good due to age.

All people of all ages have aches and pains, bladder problems, bowel problems, heart problems - problems remembering, even at the high school level. But you can learn to manage your health, so that you will be able to perform daily tasks in a most efficient way, second to none.

One of my clients made a thought provoking statement. "If a person just died when they got sick that might be okay. But I see people get sick and then for the next twenty years or more they live a life of continuing, progressively worse illnesses, with unbearable pain and misery. I don't want to do that, so I am going to do all I can to get healthy and stay there." In prevention, an example is the way ascorbate keeps the bladder healthy.

This report covers all the ways that we have used in our own recovery as well as those we know or know about. It is the result of researching a vast store of knowledge over many years and by many researchers and scientists.   It is meant as a guide and as a *"whetting of your appetite"* in the quest for good health and quality of life. Sometimes families do not understand and neither do doctors nor friends - BUT you regain or maintain your health and that is what counts!   Others may come along later after they see your success. Sometimes well meaning friends will cut out articles from newspapers to show you that you are taking the wrong things. Others will show you articles that tell that someone died from taking what you are taking.

TV talk shows and news reports often tell negative things about health supplements. Bear in mind that any such reports are based on partial information making them false. A half truth is a lie. One is wise to find out who is funding the sources of information. From that knowledge base you can determine whether or not you will allow it into your reasoning.

There is a view held by many that much 'research' has been   commissioned specially to achieve a required result which either changes a public perception or is designed to maintain a state of confusion to which many people admit. The constant 'to and fro' of the arguments for and against the importance of dietary cholesterol and even blood cholesterol, are examples that have both driven food choices and also maintained confusion.

One must remember that more often than not, radical treatments or treatments given too late actually caused the death, even though the person tried to help himself by natural means. Remember also, that typically 10% of what you read In the newspaper is true.

That means 90% of the rest is edited and full of the opinions of the persons writing the article. They are often very biased and certainly not people you would want to trust to find your way to a balanced and healthy life. In fact, I would like to do a consultation for such journalists to assess their health and lifestyle.

It is really up to each of us to take control of our own health and do all of which we are made aware, to help in this pursuit. The more we know the better base we have for making choices and decisions. We do have a right to choose our health care. To receive a *"thank you"* from my client is an extra bonus. Just feeling good from day to day as I go about my activities - teaching others how to regain or maintain a healthy and balanced life, full of vigor and vitality is its own reward.

Skeletal System Health
For bone health it is important for you to eliminate all aluminum products including cookware, aluminum foil wrap for cooking food, antiperspirant deodorants, and antacids containing aluminium from your lifestyle, as well as some cosmetics. Again let me repeat, if you have indigestion, you can take enzymes to help digest the food rather than waiting for an acid condition to develop from undigested foods, sending the burning sensation up your esophagus.

In addition to aluminum these products contain too much phosphorus and upset the balance of calcium in the bones, which can result in aches and pains. Depending on your age and sex, you most likely need calcium supplements daily, along with a balance of magnesium. They should be in equal milligrams rather than having an imbalance of calcium over magnesium. Chocolate of course, will rob your body of the ability to use calcium correctly. This is old knowledge passed on from my mother and is now being taught by major health care professionals all across America. Remember, you don't really like chocolate, unless you enjoy eating it without any trace of sugar! It is the sugar that people crave!

Hair loss:
Abnormal falling of hair can be prevented or re-grown by taking *PABA 100mg, Biotin 100 mg, Folic Acid 500 mcg, and Inositol 100mg* daily for two or three weeks then decreasing to half. Continue until hair ceases to fall. If your deficiency is severe it may take six months to restore your nutritional needs of these vitamins. (Adelle Davis *Let's Get Well*, P. 138 139.) I have seen this formula turn around the hair loss to a full head of thick hair. The actual strands of hair became thicker as they grew out of the scalp.

Immune System Response:
Gluconic DMG is excellent for building one's immune response by as much as 400%. This has been shown to be true in both human and animal studies. Besides helping suppressed immune systems, it increases circulation, oxygen utilization, glucose metabolism, neurological function, and cardiovascular health.

Another product by Standard Process, *Immuplex* is an excellent immune system builder. *Bee propolis* is also a powerful immune booster, protecting against all kinds of invaders that can destroy health and well being. It is a fine powder and tastes something like chocolate when mixed into Rice "Milk" or Almond Breeze. The bees gather it from tree bark and buds. They use it to disinfect their hives, among other things. All bees must walk through this Propolis before entering the hive. All enemies that have been killed, but are too large to remove from the hive, are covered with *Propolis* and they never rot. *Grapefruit Extract* and Olive Leaf Extract are other helpers from nature that will boost us over infections of all kinds. Many companies provide products that combine a number of ingredients that will help the immune system. Some include Raw Thymus and other glandulars, along with herbs and other nutrients.

Lacrimal gland

One would not normally relate the Lacrimal gland to the immune system so it may come as a surprise to learn that part of the function of this gland is to provide a service to the blood and the eye by taking in oxidised or 'spent Vitamin C, dehydroascorbic acid (DHAA) from the circulation reducing it and delivering the product to the anterior surface of the eye. Now we need to know how fish protect their cornea.

Low Back Pain

First and foremost, any joint pain must have the right nutrients to keep the connective tissue, synovial fluid and collagen healthy so that bone does not rub on bone. Hyaluronic Acid, Chondroitin, Glucosamine and MSM are your major line of defense to relieve pain in any joint whether back or knees, elbows, shoulders, wrists ankles, etc. And don't forget your healthy oils!

So many people, who have had illnesses associated with heavy lifting or surgeries, complain of low back pain. For lighter cramps or stiffness you experience, you can find a stretching position that will release the tension on those muscles before they go into spasms.

Some people bend forward and try to touch their toes, gently bouncing until the hands almost touch the floor. For others the tension causing the pain is the other way and lying down across the bed on the back will stretch those muscles the other way for relief. Find what works for you and use it consistently to reduce tension built up in the muscles.

Few realise how Optometrists suffer particularly, holding their posture for ophthalmoscopy. Sometimes a cold compress will relieve the pain by reducing inflammation. Pain usually indicates inflammation. When the area is cold the body will automatically flood that area with a fresh supply of blood bringing with it the nutrients needed for healing.

Dr Laurie Plaisance-Ross, DC recommends warm applications saying "We are warm blooded creatures." Warm is more relaxing but if there is inflammation in the area it will cause more irritation and accelerated pain, especially in the joints.

Wearing an elastic back support can give relief, but excessive use causes the muscles to atrophy rather than strengthen to support your back in a healthy posture. A study for home improvement stores, showed that employees should limit wearing elastic back supports, releasing the tension except when they need to lift, similar to the support that weight lifters give their bodies when they lift, using a kidney belt.

It was determined that wearing the belt tight all the time, would weaken the muscles rather than strengthen them. The support was needed to help with lifting so the back would not be compromised. Statistics for back injury shows a high correlation to absenteeism in the work place.

Walking and swimming are the most wonderful low back builders, because they do not put lifting stress on the low back area. Wrestler's Press builds the low back. Lie flat on the floor. Raise knees up so that the heels touch the buttocks. Now press the hips up toward the ceiling as far as possible, and hold a couple seconds. Release to the floor and repeat, gradually increasing the number of your repetitions.

Cold and hot compresses (fomentations) to the painful area often bring relief. This is done by using a hand towel dipped and wrung out from a basin of hot water. Then after six minutes it is replaced with another towel for one minute that has been dipped in cold water and wrung out. If repeated three times in a row, it will often bring great relief from pain without the use of any drugs.

Back pain can also be directly connected to bowel irregularity, so be sure to check yourself on that. If uncertain, you probably need to increase your Vitamin C intake or a good herbal laxative and a continuing vigilance in that department. A thorough cleansing of the bowel through the use of a tissue cleansing diet and colon cleansing program, will often give complete relief from back pain.

For "arthritis like" pain in hip joints, knees, elbows or back, the warm, dry heat application may offer the most effective relief. Skilled acupuncture work with the meridians of energy known by Chinese and Japanese people for centuries before western medicine came into being are very effective. Dr Bush has described incredible personal experiences when Western Medicine has failed him. In some cases

Proteolytic Enzymes are a very effective anti-inflammatory. They need to be taken 3 to 5 capsules at a time on an empty stomach with a large glass of water, as an anti-inflammatory to relieve pain.

White Willow Bark is a wonderful pain reliever. Pharmaceutically, the salicylic acid in willow bark is chemically synthesized and produced in large quantities to make aspirin. This aspirin causes blood loss in the stomach and leaky gut in the bowels whereas willow bark, with the salicylic acid in its natural state has no side effect. It must be taken over time and builds its effectiveness gradually, whereas aspirin works faster but has deleterious effects on the body. One side effect of the use of NSAID's is leaky gut which results in more food allergies. Before long one wonders "Now what is going wrong with my body?"

You can take 2 capsules for pain relief every 3 hours. Also *Feverfew,* (2 capsules) is another pain relieving herb. There are various sport rubs that help relieve these types of pain and are applied to the skin. *ArthriGel* by Gero-Vita is also very good. Another topical application for pain in the joints is *Tiger Balm,* a Chinese product and available in most health food stores. It should not be used if you are taking homeopathic remedies as it will cancel their effect. Anything with camphor or strong essential oils, falls into this same category. *Arnica Montana* oil is excellent massage oil for pain or injuries. Topical application of this oil will almost always give instant relief from pain. *Emu Oil* is effective for pain also and has a wonderful soothing effect on the skin, if there is any soreness, etc.. It is a 'driver' and will carry other applications into the body for greater relief. We cannot leave this discussion without mentioning DMSO as a pain relief agent. It must be applied in short dabs rather than rubbed into the skin because it will create a very uncomfortable burning sensation like oil of wintergreen.

Believe it or not, lack of exercise can cause joint and back pains, because the muscles lose their strength when not used. We call it atrophy of the muscles. Then the stress of weight bearing is put on the joints which should be supported by the muscles.

Note: Dependence on back supports can contribute to a weakening of the muscles in the back so care needs to be taken if one is worn at your work place. Alternate so that you wear it tight only when lifting.

Walking is inexpensive and quite easy. You should aim to build up to three miles every other day or 1 ½ miles per day. Swimming is excellent, too. You could take a Detoxosode from your health care professional, to rid the body of chlorine after swimming. A detoxosode is designed to help your body release toxins. You can also wash your hair with shampoo that cleanses it of chlorine. Be sure to ask your Homeopath for this type product if you are going to swim in chlorinated water. Perhaps we will be able to make changes in how our water is purified, using non-toxic ozone rather than chlorine, as they do in Germany and some American cities. Fluoride of course is very toxic.

You are fortunate, if you have your own re-bounder. That gives you some very good aerobic exercise while assisting your immune system as well. The immune system has no pump of its own as the circulatory system does. Little re-bounders can be set up in an office, bedroom or living room and used whenever you have a few minutes.

When we rebound or jump, as on a small trampoline, we help the lymph glands pump out toxins. If you have a treadmill that would also help as far as exercise goes. Probably the time constraints will be the most challenging for your exercise program. It is a must for good health and a healthy metabolism to use your food correctly rather than storing it as extra weight to carry around.

Don't give up just because you are not always faithful to your exercise program. Keep that goal in front of you - regular exercises! Office jobs make this a real challenge, so discipline is required. Keep in mind that it is for your health to feel better afterward.

Laughter
Yes "laughter does good like a medicine" the Bible says. Norman Cousins, in his battle against cancer, rented a lot of Laurel and Hardy movies and literally laughed himself well. He also took mega doses of Vitamin C, which contributed immensely to his survival. Try to look at things that are lovely, listen to pleasant music that inspires you and makes you happy. Don't listen to people who give you a "no hope" answer for your health concerns. In summary; All the following factors must be operational for good balanced health and eye nutrition.

Air
Clean air is essential to health. Deep breathing is paramount to getting oxygen into the alveoli where gas exchange takes place. Without air we would be dead in a few minutes. Brain and heart damage occur very rapidly without sufficient oxygen yet we often spend a whole lifetime with shallow breathing and lazy physical activity that does not require us to breathe deeply.

Water

Water must be purified to make sure there is no chlorine or other chemical that would clog up the liver and other bodily processes. We are made mostly of water so it behoves us to make sure it is good water. There is a multitude of types of filtered and processes available, which include reverse osmosis, carbon filters, and Kangen water, etc., then, by study, one learns how complicated and important it is.

Ascorbate also purifies water.

It is interesting that ascorbic acid kills pathogens in drinking water in low concentration. Less than 1% is needed. Ascorbate will substitute for ascorbic acid.

Food

Use organic food when possible. For vegetable and fruits one should always wash thoroughly, to eliminate parasites, viruses and bacteria. If one cannot obtain organically grown foods, it is imperative for good health that one washes them thoroughly to remove all waxes and chemical sprays. Peel should be removed and melons should not be eaten too close to the rind to avoid chemicals.

Body Exercises

Make sure you get enough exercise. There are a lot of easy plans where they say you do not have to exercise for good health. But our bodies are made to move and when they become inactive that is when toxins and fat cells can settle into areas where action is less. Jack La Lane used to say that the American trademark was "love handles", (fat deposits at the waist toward the back) showing that people do not bend and stretch but ride wherever they go and use machinery and elevators to do the most elemental exercise.

Supplements

Be sure to check the sources of all supplements to make sure they contain what they advertise. Those that are chemically synthesized are often not bioavailable and therefore least effective. They should be free of excipients and made from organically grown foods and animals whenever possible. I only know three companies who claim these standards, i.e., Standard Process Labs, Premier Research Labs and Dr Shultze. Da Vinci Labs and Progressive Labs are family businesses and their products are produced on FDA approved facilities though not always from organically grown foods. I am just acquiring more knowledge of others that are aimed toward Eye Nutrition but do not have a complete list at this time. One is ZeaVision and the other Life Extension (USA). Use supplements preferably with the guidance of a Clinical Nutritionist or a doctor who practices Complementary Medicine (an MD who also uses Nutrition) or Alternate Therapy Medicine such as NDs or NMD's.

If you try to self diagnose you may run into more problems than you had originally. A trained professional will know the correct dose for any given condition and will be able to direct you to the laboratories that get the best results from their products. They cannot be guided by market hype because their products must do what they claim or as you would expect, doctors will no longer order from them.

Sleep

Make sure you get restful sleep. During those hours your body is busy repairing, replacing and replenishing. Make that sleep time about 8 hours per 24 hour period. Sleep conserves your vitamin C and should be supplemented with enough Lysine either from meat, fish, eggs, milk or cheese or a Lysine supplement. Without Lysine the sleep/rest period cannot complete the repairs needed for the cardiovascular system.

Effects of chemical drugs

Try not to take any chemical drugs. They deplete your vitamin C. That is probably why aspirin has been withdrawn as a recommendation for the prevention of thrombosis. Aspirin destroys vitamin C. Ask your doctor to wean you off all that are not needed for life. Most have serious side effects which can be worse than the original condition. Your doctor will be glad to help you, but if not you can change doctors to one who will. People who are chemically sensitive, allergic or have other sensitivities should be especially careful.

Lighting:

According to Dr Glen Welman, OD, of Estes Park, Colorado, the two colors in neon lighting are more conducive to eye health and comfort than a single color, due to the single wave length. He told us that the single color lights will cause a flickering that accelerates ocular fatigue. Such lights are mostly used in schools and super markets and cause fatigue in those who must work under them. Due to our own daughter's rapid increased myopia when she studied at a school requiring all students to study for long periods within a cubicle, illuminated by a single color neon bulb, we actually contacted Dr Welman to have his views confirmed directly to us.

He had studied students who worked in cubicles illuminated with neon bulbs and found greater eye fatigue and vision problems developing in those students than those working at desks in open conditions with incandescent overhead lighting. Also considered was the accommodation of those who working in the enclosed cubicle environment couldn't relax. He believed that was not good for the students, especially at an age when they were still developing.

Posture and distance
How often must parents warn children to move away from televisions? Children will inch up ever closer to such screens. Increasing myopia is also a worry with long use of miniature, hand held screens.
Turn on the TV. Turn off the lights. Close your eyes
Note the flickering especially with the TV commercials.
I was informed by Dr Welman that 72% of our energy is committed to vision and when that is constantly bombarded with stimuli we tire. In the UK, for the benefit of epileptics, viewers are warned when scenes will include flash photography.

Time (Eye Strain)
Working at the computer screen, or spending long hours staring at the flickering TV screen should be carefully monitored for vision health. In the US the public is warned to, read for 20 minutes, and then look away 20 feet, for 20 seconds to reduce eye strain. All other hand held devices should be used with discretion. This includes "texting" on cell phones; iPods; iPads; Smart phones, Androids and other small, backlit reading surfaces such as the Nook and Kindle readers, although these readers allow for larger type fonts, there are still the backlit surface that may affect vision if good viewing practices are not observed

Chapter II.
Specific Nutrition for Vision Problems (Without its many references to the Internet this section would be massive!)

The scope of this book cannot match those published in many volumes. It is necessary to omit much content of a degree course in Nutrition. This, forming part of the course for the planned professional doctorate in CardioRetinometry, a further work will deal in greater depth e.g., with Bioflavonoids, antioxidants, and additional eye diseases.

The synergistic action of vitamins C and E needs emphasis and the way in which bioflavonoids potentiate them is essential knowledge. Similarly, mitochondria, the biological clock for your biological age will be omitted with specific mitochondrial antioxidants our knowledge of which we attribute to Denham Harman.

It being impossible to address every ocular condition, the most important are addressed. In this way it is hoped to keep the interest of the reader and make learning more interesting. Churchill said "Everyone likes learning. Few like being taught."

Musculo-skeletal problems such as an ocular torticollis, are not strictly in the purview of this book, but it would be very incomplete if we were to omit the 'classical' and dramatic experience of Norman Cousins, former editor of the *Saturday Review*. Described by him in his book *Anatomy of an Illness as Perceived by the Patient,* he relates how, with severe arthritis culminating in Ankylosing Spondylitis, he discharged himself from hospital in order to be

Injected with 35 grams of ascorbate daily in a hotel bedroom by his own physician and was cured.

Below are lists of ingredients thought to help or have been shown in studies or by actual experience, to benefit vision and to increase circulation to the eye and brain.

MRSA Infection
This is the best place to include a treatment for keratitis that is banned in the UK. Gut Sod. Ascorbate were withdrawn years ago. They are specific for MRSA and Pseudomonas Aeruginosa corneal ulcer. What can anyone think of the morality of that? To their credit the British Medical Journal published a rapid response to Biant that states Nakanishi in Japan found that burns were cleared of MRSA with a sod ascorbate spray.

Please notice the sources of these ingredients. Many close their minds when one mentions herbs and immediately dismiss everything else the author says, to quackery. That makes me smile. Our herbs and their benefits will be here a thousand years after our current medicines have been withdrawn and abandoned.

Vitamin C will still work against bacteria and viruses long after new drugs have gone. So with an open mind we examine the following with food sources or descriptions.

Lutein
These extremely important carotenoids are obtained from green vegetables such as kale, spinach, turnip greens, collard greens, romaine lettuce, broccoli, zucchini and Brussels sprouts

Lutein absorption
Its absorption is enhanced when spinach is served with eggs because it is fat soluble and needs the fats in egg yolk as our grandparents seemed to know. www.whfoods.org Zeaxanthin, another carotenoid, is also included in these foods. Its bioavailability is high in tomatoes, as well as papaya and watermelon.

Neo-Zeaxanthin
This is a third type of xanthophyll and may help to reduce fatty build up in the arteries along with Lutein, Zeaxanthin , Vit C, Vit E and Omega 3 fatty acids. to benefit the heart as well as vision, so says Dr Heiting of www.allaboutvision.com. This is in total agreement with Dr Bush's theory and protocol.

Lycopene
Well known as an antioxidant with high concentrations in Tomatoes, watermelon and papaya www.Livestrong.com

Bilberry (vaccinium myrtillus)
has a high concentration anthosianaside antioxidants, catechins, lutein, and tannins which can protect against free radicals. It is rich in a number of nutrients that are specific to the eyes, supports healthy capillaries, collagen production, and protects against cell damage. Balch, Phyllis A. "Prescription for Nutritional Healing,4th Ed., (Penguin Books 2006) http://necam.nih.gov/health/bilberry/

L-Arginine, is an amino acid found in higher concentrations in red meats, nuts and seeds such as pumpkin and squash. Sporadically in a few different foods, including tofu, whole-grain wheat flour, garlic, onions and chocolate syrup.

Green Tea
deserves a special mention. It is a good source of antioxidants and alkaloids. It contains various vitamins like A, D, E, C, B, B5, H and K. and is a rich source of Manganese as well as Zinc, Chromium and

Selenium.
The most important active component in green tea epigallocatechin-3-gallate (EGCG) is a many times more powerful antioxidant than vitamin C or vitamin E alone when taken according to RDA advice.
Enagic of Japan shows studies that too much is not good. Those who drank less green tea in one study, noticed a lower incidence of colon cancer. or polyps. www.Greenteanutritionfacts.com

A further Japanese study conducted by Dr Hiromi Shinya, who invented and perfected the colonoscopy procedure so commonly used today without major surgery, found that excessive use of Green Tea was not conducive to continued health of those who had had polyps removed by this procedure. He was also the Doctor of Ronald Regan.

Gingkgo Biloba
is a very old herb, the leaf of which contains Flavoneglycosides, 6% [7.2 mg] Terpene Lactones and 0.8% [0.96 mg] Ginkgolide B) It allows nutrient to cross the blood brain barrier. This has obvious significance for the retinal circulation.

Alpha-Lipoic acid. The "Consumption of ALA from food has not yet been found to result in detectable increases of free LA in plasma or cells. In, high oral doses of free LA (≥ 50 mg) result in significant but transient increases in free acid in the plasma and cells." www.lpi.org at Oregon State University is probably the most comprehensive site for additional scientific evidence of the value of this protector of mitochondrial health.

Burt Berkson

Is a physician who, at considerable risk to his career, disobeyed hospital orders and almost lost his job. His book gives some idea of the complex functions and needs for this co-enzyme. Berkson, using only ALA, saved an elderly couple who were abandoned to die in hospital having eaten deadly toadstools. Disciplined he risked his job to save others

Functions

Prevent organ dysfunction
Reduce endothelial dysfunction and improve albuminuria. Treat or prevent cardiovascular disease
Accelerate chronic wound healing
Reduce levels of ADMA in diabetic end-stage renal disease patients on hemodialysis[
Management of burning mouth syndrome
Reduce iron overload
Treat metabolic syndrome
Improve or prevent age-related cognitive dysfunction
Prevent or slow the progression of Alzheimer's Disease
Prevent erectile dysfunction (animal models but anecdotally applies to humans as well)
Prevent migraines[
Treat multiple sclerosis
Treat chronic diseases associated with oxidative stress
Reduce inflammation
Inhibit advanced glycation end products (AGE) Treat peripheral artery disease.

Grape Seed from a fruit, contains Proanthocyanadins and "can benefit in many other ways, i.e, it can be used to prevent health problems which include cardiovascular disease, varicose veins, edema, and arthritis. An extract also acts as a natural anti-histamine, moderating allergic responses by reducing histamine production and boosting the immune system.

L-lysine
Performs a major role in the health of the eye. It is an essential amino acid, i.e., we need to take it in each day through food or supplements, because we do not make it from other proteins. It potentiates Vitamin C in its control of cholesterol, and it too must be supplied each day since we do not make our own supply of this absolutely vital nutrient.

Best sources are most all meats, nuts legumes whole eggs, whole milk and cheeses.

Meats are in the thousands of milligrams, Nuts and seeds in the hundreds of milligrams and vegetables with the exception of chick peas, garbanzo beans, green peas, asparagus, wheat germ and Lentil sprouts, which are in the category of about 300 mg per serving. No fruits make the list as a good source.

Grape seed extract is frequently recommended to combat macular degeneration, cataracts, and eye strain. Studies have shown that 300 mg daily reduces eye strain from prolonged computer use in 60 days.

Learn more:
http://www.naturalnews.com/029223_grape_seed_e
xtract_health.html#ixzz29aWdN3fE

Pycnogenols
Derived from Maritime Pine Bark from France, are another important supplement that can help These Proanthocyanadins will cause (proven in dark field microscopy) an un-clumping of blood cells for free flowing into the tiniest capillaries.

Turmeric (Curcumin) contains high antioxidants
as well as the following nutrients valuable for good health
"100 g of turmeric provides (% of RDA per 100 g):
53% dietary fiber,
138% of vitamin B-6 (pyridoxine),
32% of niacin,
43% of vitamin C,
21% of vitamin E,
54% of potassium,
517% of iron,
340%of manganese and   40 % of zinc.
www.nutrition-and-you.com

Vitamin C
All the forms of Vit C and their attributes
as listed in the Linus Pauling Institute. It must be sodium ascorbate, not synthesized from ascorbic acid with little rose hips in it, to label it "natural".
Foods that are cooked or stored for long periods of time will lose their vitamin C value. So eating fresh raw foods in recommended for highest quality, but needs to be supplemented with Vitamin C preferably in the powdered form of   Sodium Ascorbate to overcome the deficiency that most all humans experience. See 700 Vitamin C Secrets by Dr Bush

concerning the inability of humans and guinea pigs to make their own Vitamin C. producing Scurvy which is now referred to as a Vitamin Deficiency rather than the original medical term 'Scurvy.'

Food sources for Vitamin C are:
Cantaloupe
Citrus fruits and juices, such as orange and grapefruit
Kiwi fruit
Mango
Papaya
Pineapple
Strawberries, raspberries, blueberries, cranberries
Watermelon
Vegetables that are the highest sources of vitamin C include:
Italian Broad leaf Parsley
Broccoli, Brussels sprouts, cauliflower
Green and red peppers
Spinach, cabbage, turnip greens, and leafy greens
Sweet and white potatoes
Tomatoes and tomato juice
Winter squash

Although some grains also include vitamin C, most are cooked, which reduces the efficacy of this vital part vitamin and hormone.

Read more:
http://www.umm.edu/ency/article/002404fod.htm#i
xzz29ag2OUTv

Vitamin A,
This must be in a form that does not turn rancid. These are best found in raw fresh foods.
The most potent ones are dark green leafy vegetables,

carrots, sweet potatoes, Paprika, Cayenne and Chili powder as well as the old favorite which many refuse, i.e., liver. If you are averse to eating liver, desiccated liver can be taken as a supplement in a raw freeze dried tablet.

If you feel that you cannot tolerate these foods due to the feeling that your liver may not be able to handle this fat soluble vitamin, you can take the emulsified form as A-Emulsion which is how the young undeveloped liver of an infant receives it from his mother's milk. Infantile scurvy is of course, a threat.

Vitamin E MUST be *natural* the most bioavailable form; never synthetic. Sadly most all studies have been done with synthetic forms, rendering them useless as far a nutritional value is concerned.

Feverfew, an herb from the chrysanthemum family, "contains high amounts of the minerals iron, niacin, manganese, phosphorus, potassium and selenium. It also contains smaller levels of the minerals silicon, sodium and zinc. Feverfew also contains the Vitamins A and C. Parthenolide is the active ingredient in Feverfew and helps red blood cells [RBC's] to move through the smaller blood vessels in the head to maintain proper circulation and fluid balance. Feverfew contains properties that work with the body to regulate normal body function " www.DrSatnadley.com

Resveratrol, an antioxidant, is found in the skin of red grapes and in other fruits. Although the jury is still out as to long term use, the value of a natural food such as the skins of grapes can hardly be denied or refuted from any existing formal scientific study.

People have been eating grapes for much longer than modern Western medicine has been around. Resveratrol was developed by Bill Sardi and Longevinex Partners in association with Harvard University. There are great difficulties in its preparation to provide the highest potency presentation in this competitve market. With Harvard's help, Sardi brought the first and probably the best product to the public. Market America claims an isotonic form that is absorbed into the body from the stomach within 20 minutes of ingestion, as if one had an intravenous injection.

Antioxidants.
I have already covered about as many sources as can be found, at least those that are most plentiful in antioxidants, carotenoids and xanthophylls. The most valuable ones are contained in dark colored vegetables and fruits

Water soluble antioxidants of the eye have recently been evaluated by high performance liquid chromatography with electrochemical detection. According to Rose and Wilson, significant amounts of ascorbic acid (AA) (0,73 micro Moles) were found in human and rabbit aqueous humor (Richer and Rose)

Glaudulars such as Ocular PMG (Photomorphogen extract from organs or glands), can come from many different glands. This one is from bovine or porcine eye. The theory behind this is that "like heals like."

Oculatrophin contains phytonutrients from organic sources. We have a lot to learn about the value of phytonutrients often overlooked as not as vitamin and minerals in our diet.

Phytochemicals

"One of the most important groups of phytochemicals are the phytosterols or phytohormones as they are sometimes known. These are plant based sterols that act as precursors to human sterols. They act to modulate the human endocrine system. One of the most important human sterols is Dehydroepi-androsterone (DHEA).

Dehydroepi-androsterone (DHEA).

This hormone is produced in our adrenal glands and serves a variety of functions. It is often called the 'mother' hormone as it has the ability to convert itself into other hormones such as oestrogen, testosterone, progesterone, and corticosterone, on demand. Thus it is a precursor to all other hormones and active metabolites. Precursors are substances the body uses to produce other substances."
Glyconutrient website

Decline of DHEA

DHEA, declines with age from 25 and up. It has many affects such as with cancer, heart disease and even osteoporosis. It is the precursor of stress hormones such as Cortisol and adrenaline with vitamin C. That is, our body makes Cortisol and adrenaline from DHEA.

As DHEA levels decline. we may be under more stress which has debilitating effects on the body. With our stressful lives it is no wonder that most people have deficient levels of DHEA and the medical conditions, and degenerative diseases listed above.

HORMONES

Information on hormones is very important and should be tested by your health care professional rather than taking the latest popular demand hormone sold. It is not good to guess and self diagnose or medicate.

ADRENALS

Your adrenal glands are of particular importance as, they govern your flight or fright reflex as well as the circadian rhythm of sleep/wake cycles and glucose balance.

Good rest is important for adrenals to operate properly and if necessary they should be supplemented. If you are one who stays awake late and rises late you might need to reset your adrenal glands to produce the correct amount of Cortisol. That is done by supplementing Phosphatidyl serine in the evening to cut down the Cortisol, then in the morning the Cortisol can be brought back up, by nourishing the adrenals with other supplements to increase function. When this protocol is followed for two to three weeks in an effort to mimic the correct circadian rhythm, then the body will take over and do it's job and continued supplementation is unnecessary. You will need to watch your stress levels and keep good habits retiring early so Cortisol doesn't again overbalance.

In a female hormonal check for example you will find several hormones that are important to women's needs. There are also other male hormones. For the female for example the Testosterone is as important as it is for the male but in different ratios. Just as the estrogen in the form of Estrogen hormones, Estriol, Estrone, Estodial, may be dominant for the female, males also need this typically dominant female hormone in the correct amount

To summarize then, we need to use the darkest of all the vegetables and fruits in the reds and greens for the highest antioxidant content.

These include spinach and kale and many others as above. The Western world is totally brain washed about cholesterol being the cause of heart attacks although never proved that heart attack victims have high cholesterol! It isn't true. Lande & Sperry in 1936 proved it, then S.K. Mathur. The whole egg is recommended. Many have been convinced to throw away the yolk and eat the white. Although some have worried about the cholesterol in eggs, that is a needless worry since the yolk not only contains zeaxanthin and lutein which enhance the macular pigment, but also sufficient lecithin to balance the egg as a near perfect food. One wonders how many vision problems have developed using this wasteful practice of throwing away the egg yolk.

In CardioRetinometry® there is no concern with high cholesterol. Most people who have heart attacks and strokes (& 60% do!) MUST have normal cholesterol! The Brown Bear has three times as much as humans! My son's in-laws have high and low cholesterol; He has had three strokes with low cholesterol! Dr Bush's CardioRetinometry® could have prevented those strokes by monitored atherolysis. Truly man is born to extremes. When an idea is held to be true, we close our minds and deprive ourselves of necessary nutrients or overload ourselves with some good ones that are not good when overdone. More is not always better. Over and over we must learn all we can from research, and experience, but knowledge and intelligence are not wisdom. Common sense is required. This brings us to

A NEW CONCEPT OF INTRAOCULAR PRESSURE
Why isn't atheroma seen in the circumcorneal vessels? Cerebral circulation is opposed by Cerebro-Spinal Fluid Pressure (causing carotid atheroma) the IOP opposing retinal circulation, causes arteriolar reflex. (Bush). Circulation is vital. My nutrients to lower intraocular pressure reached only one eye. My CardioRetinometry programme countered this through increased cerebral circulation, not just of the eyes, but ears, and brain. With age, ocular connective tissue lost elasticity, stiffening with cross linking like an old sponge. *The optic nerve head was damaged by malnutrition, which (1) caused collapse of the trabeculum (2) then caused high IOP and (3) then collapsed atrophic neural tissue of the ONH which (4) was repairable by supplements targeting neural collagen.* Note: Dr. Bush says my glaucoma was caused by sleeping for 30 yrs face down, with my left eye pressed into the pillow, compromising the trabecular circulation and nutrition. An example: Nerve sheath healed completely in a type two diabetic who fell four times, saying "It felt like a wire in front of her leg." Neuerotrophin and Neuroplex phytonutrients, from organically grown vegetables, fruits and animals (Standard Process, Inc) recovered the

112

use of the leg. Her only western medical option was a leg brace which would not have prevented a fall.

As Dr. Bush has learned in discovering CardioRetinometry®, we do not accept the status quo or the diagnosis of "no hope". Yes we may go against the tide, but so did many others who have gone before us. We are thankful for those who think for themselves rather than become parrots of their education.

One phrase that I learned as a late teenager is "Any dead fish can float down stream but it takes a lively one to swim against the current to reach its destination". Dr Walter Kneble told us in the mid sixties, that "It is the younger doctors who will make the changes necessary for good health because they are not yet brain washed."

The following ingredients have been shown to increase circulation to the head, enhance mental clarity and focus attention. None of them is caffeine based so can be safely used for those with IOP concerns. It behooves us in the health field to take care of our own brains so that we an continue to offer the best of the best in health care.

DMAE (Dimethylaminoethanol)
Alpha GPC (Glycerolphosphorylcholine)
PS (Phosphatidylserine) long known to decrease Cortisol when a person is. undergoing adrenal stress, but, is also a powerful neurotransmitter so increase the circulation to the brain and head in general.

Gotu Kola has been in use for 3,000 years as a medicinally valued plant. This grand old herb contains no caffeine but many other useful constituents such as asiaticoside (a triterpene glycoside) (triterpenoid and sesquiterpene), brahmoside and brahminoside (both saponin glycosides), madecassoside (a glycoside with strong anti-inflammatory properties), madecassic acid, thiamine, riboflavin, pyridoxine, vitamin K, aspartate, glutamate, serine, threonine, alanine, lysine, histidine, magnesium, calcium and msodiu.

Guarana contains caffeine and should not be used by those with cardiac issues, high blood pressure or Glaucoma without the specific direction of your health care professional because of its stimulating effects.

Guarana (Paullinia Cupana) is from the soap berry family. Its seeds are made into a paste. The main use of this herb is for its energy effects. Its crystalline principle is said to be identical to caffeine. It also contains tannins. Its use is medicinal and for food; candy, soft drinks and the highly esteemed Guarana bread. It also has antioxidant properties and is used as a mental stimulant, to increase libido, central nervous system stimulant, and enhance athletic performance. Do not use to cover up physical symptoms not diagnosed by your doctor. Oxford Dictionary, London, 1979 and http://www.webmd/.

Lutein alone and in combination with Zeaxanthin and Neo-Zeaxanthin benefit not only eye health but the cardiovascular system. Since 1992 there are many ongoing studies to prove the efficacy of these valuable antioxidants and ascorbate. The fovea of the eye in particular contains a high ratio of these nutrients

Bioperine (black pepper) Bioperine is an alkaloid found in black pepper. Studies show that when bioperine is taken with supplements there is an increase by 60% of the nutrients. Absorbed in the intestines. (www.Dr Ricketsnutri.com)

"Huperzine A is derived from Chinese Club Moss." It helps "keep your acetylcholine levels up, so your synapses fire fast and efficiently," improves memory, and protects from "excitotoxicity." 20/20 Brain Power, Joseph Reynolds, p. 122

Cautiously, I would mention that this is being trialled to reverse neuro-disorders like Alzheimer's, especially in China. Calcium is necessary for bone and muscle health and is best absorbed when taken from food rather than ground up rock. It should be taken with the proper ratios of our vitamin D3 and Magnesium.

Ginkgo Biloba "Laboratory studies have shown that ginkgo improves blood circulation by dilating blood vessels and reducing the stickiness of blood platelets.".. .as reported by the University Of Maryland Medical Center. Read more: http://www.umm.edu/altmed/articles/ginkgo-biloba-000247.htm#ixzz29sehEDaK

Phosphorus "The Linus Pauling Institute supports the RDA for phosphorus (700 mg/day for adults). Although few multivitamin/mineral supplements contain more than 15% of the current RDA for phosphorus, a varied diet should easily provide adequate phosphorus for most people." www. Linus Pauling Institute of Oregon State University.org

Feverfew is an Aperient (a gentle purgative) , carminative; a parthenolide which may decrease the chemicals that cause migraines. It is effective in relieving pain due to eye strain because of its ability to render smooth muscle cells less responsive to body chemicals that trigger muscle spasms. Thus it becomes an effective eye nutrient especially for those who spend long hours at that computer.

"Vinpocetine is a man-made chemical resembling a substance found in the periwinkle plant Vinca minor." It is thought to enhance blood flow to the brain and is thus used for conditions that could harm learning, memory, and information processing as people age.

N-Acetyl L-Carnosine:
When administered topically to the eye in the form of N-acetyl-L-carnosine-(functionally, a time-release form of carnosine), this dipeptide can move easily into both the water-soluble (aqueous) and lipid (fat)-containing parts of the eye. Once there, it helps to prevent DNA strand breaks induced by UV radiation and enhances DNA repair. Once it has entered the lipid areas of the eye, N-acetyl-L-carnosine partially breaks down and becomes L carnosine (Life Extension USA)

Astaxanthin
is the most powerful carotenoid antioxidant and, like vitamin C, crosses the blood brain barrier. It is Lipid soluble so requires the good oils to become bioavailable. It is a naturally, creating its own protection against UV Rays when its water source is not available.

Blueberry vs Bilberry
Blueberry Eye Health Benefits
Blueberries are high in antioxidant value so are certainly to be added to an antioxidant diet. At present I was unable to find clinical trials that prove

their validity as to eye health. Here we would need to rely on anecdotal evidence and common sense.

Bilberry Eye Health Benefits
Optometrists and Nutritionists are dismayed by excessive claims targeted at our patients for eye related nutrient benefits. I am sure that if eyeglasses are e.g. 0.75 too weak, such claims are invalid. But only qualified nutritionists (NOT OPTOMETRISTS!) can persuade patients of this!

There is some truth in the following, e.g. "Bilberry's health benefits are known. Recent work shows bilberry reducing computer related strain, protecting against glaucoma, and maintaining blood vessel integrity. It reduces cataract risk, stabilizes connective tissue and reduces diabetic retinopathy." The Eye Health Centre website summed.

DMAE Dimethylaminoethanol)
can be found in fish such as salmon, sardines, anchovies and pilchards.. It is found in the brain in small quantities promoting the production of choline, a chief neurotransmitter for memory, focus and attention. More ascorbate is found of course.

Alpha GPC (Glycerolphosphorylcholine) is
the chemical precursor to acetylcholine. Derived from soy lecithin it has been used successfully to restore memory function in Stroke and Alzheimer's patients.

Phosphatidyl serine
The highest concentrations are found in bovine brain, Atlantic Mackerel, Chicken heart, Atlantic herring and

Eel. It is a strong neurotransmitter assisting in the transmission of signals cross the synapses in the brain It is also a Cortisol managing supplement.

Celandine
This product can be obtained from iHerb as a Liquid extract.

As an added help I enter this formula for Celandine by Dr Edward E. Shook, my instructor in *Advanced Herbology* (page 289.) I have used it personally for this purpose with great success.
Celandine (Chelidonium majus) Formula to dissolve viscous tears that interfere with clear vision. One formula is for infusion as in making tea. The other is a decoction and must be boiled and strained for a concentrated solution and consequently a lower dose is required than of the infusion.

Infusion
Ingredients:
One ounce Celandine herb (cut)
A pint and a quarter (20 ounces) of distilled water.
Process 1:
Bring the water to boil
Place herbs in water
Cover and remove from heat
Steep 3-5 minutes
Strain and pour into a container from which you will dispense it.

Process 2:
 Add to this infusion, one (1) ounce of glycerin and four (4) ounces of un-strained un-heated honey.
Dosage is one ounce three times per day between meals. Serve hot. Warning: Do not give to children.

The dosage needs to be governed according to bowel tolerance so that a watery stool is not produced. If that happens, cut back to find the right dose.

Decoction
The decoction is much stronger, adding potassium chloride and boiling down, letting stand and boiling again before final boiling, straining and bottling. The dosage is only one teaspoon (whereas an infusion dose is one ounce) A decoction is much more concentrated. I think for our purposes the Infusion will be sufficient.

Cerebral circulation
From the above mentioned nutrients that help eye health and those that improve circulation to the head, we can see there is much repetition. Let's take notice!

These are drastic to keep a healthy head which is the hard drive, so to speak, of our lives. To save one's mind and one's eyes is drastic. To be threatened with Alzheimer's or blindness is not welcomed by any of us and is often an underlying cause of dread or fear of old age. We don't even like the word "Old," because it so often calls up visions of decline.

Eye drops
Various kinds of eye drops for dry eye, allergy eyes and computer eye strain are available. Look for those that do not have preservatives in them. The Similisan line is good, especially if you are dealing with a patient who has allergies or sensitivities. Dr Bush also recommends Vitamin C 5% eye drops but 'dry eye' is very possibly a sign of low vitamin C! These are now

unobtainable in the UK, presumably because they threaten antihistamine and antibiotic medications. Elizabeth Baker, a nutritionist, recommends pure honey, dropped into the eye to clear infection. It acts as an antibiotic because no germs can live in it. Pure honey has been found in the great pyramid tombs of Egypt.

Eye drops that have been shown to help with cataract formations would be worthwhile looking into if the cataract is not too far advanced. They come under various names, but the ingredients must include N Acetyl Carnosine. Used over a period of three to six months, it has been shown to reduce the opacity of the lenses, making vision less clouded. Other formulations can be procured from a compounding pharmacist and should include DMSO. It stings a little but clears the lenses. (Dr Owen's newsletter contains the formula.)

Eye washes such as used in eye cups, must be made of distilled water and the eye cups must be sterilized for each use to avoid transfer of any bacteria or virus into the eye. This is of limited value though, because of the resident bacteria on the skin and eyelids. Nutrition to strengthen the skin and eye tissue is most important for the terrain. As advised by Adelle Davis, it is the tissue health that prevents bacterial invasions and consequent infection. The pH must be 7 to 7.5 for that solution. Glycerine is a valid carrier in eye drop formulations, and many formulas add alcohol as a sanitizing agent which may cause a little sting.

CardioRetinometry®
Now for the frosting on the cake for this course, in addition to the other elements for this degree, that Dr Bush seeks to provide. These are my supplements.

for the CardioRetinometry® protocol. to increase the heart health, as proposed by Dr Bush, which he has observed many times over a long period of time and many patients, in making this great discovery.
The higher does of vitamin C are also recommended to help with many eye conditions, such as glaucoma

CardioRetinometry® protocol

Vitamin C to bowel tolerance: (also relieves stress)
Suggested to start low and increase usually to 10 gr /day up to 20 or much more in some cases depending on the condition and the individual.
Vitamin E (Natural) 1,000 iu/day
Vitamin D 3, 4,000 iu/day
Lysine 3-6 gms/day
Alpha-Lipoic Acid, 100 mgs/day (2 hours apart from Lysine 500mg
CoQ10, 100 – 500mg/day depending on age , etc.
Selenium, 200 mcg/day (micro NOT Milligrams!)
Ginkgo Biloba extract from 6 gms of leaf
Eat plenty greens, meat, fish , eggs, milk and cheese

Avoid PUFAs and Margarines

In his book *700 Vitamin C Secrets*, Dr Bush outlines all the pertinent information as a basis for CardioRetinometry®. This amazing encyclopedia is the work of one person who discovered, along with those who have gone before him, the importance of Vitamin C as related to many disease conditions in the human body. He goes beyond and names each specific condition, so that doctors, as well as the general public, can help themselves when often times there is no help in organized western medical protocols. And no small wonder, for many doctors, concerned with making a good living, do not care to take the time to study the history of their own profession much less new discoveries that are taking place before their very eyes.

In addition to vitamin C, he recommends other nutrients that work together, synergistically, to clear the intraluminal plaque from the vessels in the eye, thereby preventing strokes and heart attacks for those who follow his protocol. Your retinal photos will reveal your non-compliance if you do not follow his plan, because the predicted results will not appear.

He designs a special regimen around a health history questionnaire for each patient so that each one will have the best possible chance of success, monitoring progress to 'fine tune' the prescription. Before CardioRetinometry®, and without testing urine for vitamin C constantly, it was impossible to be certain whether or not one had been suffering from scurvy in any of a multitude of diseases.

The weird thing is that one can, very deceptively, feel perfectly well with only a half of the optimal level of vitamin C in the plasma. This will then assuredly, lead to continuous, growth of the obstructions in our heart blood vessels that eventually kill us. Indeed, that appears to have been the fate of the good doctor Hugh Riordan MD, who is said to have suddenly fallen down whilst standing at his photocopier.

When Dr. Riordan lost all his plasma vitamin C after being bitten by the spider, he was completely unaware of it. Until the daily measurements of his plasma vitamin C, which were being carried out coincidentally for other research revealed what had happened, he simply did not know the danger he was in. The trick – as Dr Matthias Rath was first to point out, is to stop the growth and better still – to keep it regressing if only by 2% or 3% per annum. This is about the current limit of photometric evaluation with ordinary cameras.

Chapter III
Common Eye Diseases

(Eye disease possibly improved or eliminated with the CardioRetinometry® protocol and higher doses of Vitamin C are found in the foregoing chapters.)

(Referral recommendations in this book relate to UK NHS protocols)

Here again, we must go back to good nutrition first and foremost, to address any health condition. Food is more easily assimilated than chemically synthesized vitamins, or ground up rock for minerals. Plants take the soil and form from it the nutrients that we can assimilate when eaten in plant and animal forms.

As a basis for many health conditions, Davis' Anti Stress Formula in her book, *Let's Get Well* (p. 329) added various vitamins and minerals for specific eye conditions. Using this as a base, we will investigate other nutrients that can be taken for the eyes. We know the value of the antioxidants and vitamin C for eye health. Again quoting Dr Hedahl here, "Whatever is good for the heart is also good for the eyes." We will not be covering the western medical drugs and surgeries for eye diseases, as valuable as they may be in some cases, rather we will stress the nutrients that help vision, and prevent problems before they arise, or at least work toward reversing some that have begun to manifest. in annual visits to your Optometrist. Davis lacked knowing that PUFAs produced Harman's 'Free Radicals,' and perhaps contributed to retinitis, but noted that these new oils worrying her, seemed to create 'softer' less stable fat.

Recent research found new antioxidants and their application to the conditions that need them.

Prolonged stress will take its toll, but one can also look to organizational, psychological, and mental strategies and skills to manage stress. Some situations demand stress, so we are not asking you to drop out of the world of challenges, but rather to prepare yourselves for the requirements of a highly productive life, that will benefit mankind. My motto "May this world be a better place when I leave than when I arrived."

Life Extension (USA), also recommends complete nutrition as a base for eye health, via their formulation "Life Extension Mix. "

In addition there are specific nutrients that address certain eye conditions. The greatest of these are antioxidants. More specifically, vitamin C and A are always first and foremost on the list of requirements.

Meal Replacement
I shouldn't pick one supplier of many with little to choose between them, but might make an exception and say that Progressive Labs in Texas supplies nutrients for the day as well. Other companies may make such formulations, but watch to make sure that they can be used as a total meal replacement Other Labs such as DaVinci of Vermont have total nutrition needs in tablet form, with the exception of L-Lysine Their formula is taken 3 or 4 times per day. There are many supplements now that can be used to replace meals and can be included in one's daily regimen to make sure that total nutrition is obtained. I recommend only one meal per day ever be replaced by this method.

Let's take a look at glaucoma for instance.

Glaucoma is a mysterious disease, hypothesised to result from high intraocular pressure. But it may be that the real cause is scorbutic. This could cause both its vascular and ocular hypertension features with collapse of the trabeculum as suggested by Bietti in 1966, and the visible optic nerve atrophy. Reversible ischemia of the ONH presumably resulting from human congenital anascorbemia (Irwin Stone) has been demonstrated by Dr. Bush in hundreds of cases.

Any and every Optometrist is expected to be able to replicate this reversal of ONH ischemia by time lapse retinal photography with vitamin C within 3 months, in almost every case where extra vitamin C has never been taken.

When a person is diagnosed with Primary Open Angle Glaucoma (POAG) as I was, with Optic Nerve Head damage already evident I was highly motivated to find an answer. Here is what I did. I searched far and wide in several different nutritional laboratories. At this point in time, my Optometrist just told me last week, "Given what you are doing, your eyes are good for another 20 years." I had to control myself from jumping off his exam chair and shouting !Hallelujah! "

Most vitamin companies have an answer for almost everything, but do have particular formulas that really work. All supplements in every company do not necessarily work for everything they are purported to help. For example, you can ask various labs what to do for any given condition and the answer might be different from lab to lab depending on their particular

125

method of production, philosophy of healing, the sources of their raw materials, your diagnosis, knowledge, treatment, and healing times. I chose a company that had great experience with life extension and anti-aging. Other labs stress organics; no excipients; production from foods or pharmaceutical grade vitamins, etc. Those all have their place in healing. Look for the ones that are most bioavailable.

Life Extension (USA) recommended for my high IOP, the following protocol, which I followed as exactly as possible, reducing my IOP by my next appointment with my Optometrist. Some I ordered and some I had in my inventory already. This is what I took to reduce IOP significantly from 29 and 32 to 18 and 18. At one appointment it was as low as 15. I am still vigilant to keep the IOP in the normal range, and working closely with my Optometrist to maintain that.

~ Eye Drops with N-Acetyl Carnosine: This was to address possible cataracts at my age.
~ Life Extension Mix : A tablespoon of powder per day
~ Vitamin C crystals to establish healthy collagen, working up to 12 grams per day according to personal bowel tolerance.
~ Proanthocyanadins from Grape skin and seed extract and French Maritime Pine Bark 150 to 300 mg daily
~ Bilberry 100 mg twice daily
~ Selenium 200 mcg daily
~ Vitamin A 12,000 to 50,000 IU per day, depending on your personal condition. Emulsified A is easier for the liver to process.
Pregnant women should consult with their health care professional.

Vitamin A increases the visual purple for night vision

as well as relieving dry itchy eyes (Where there has been a deficiency).
~ Coleus Forskolii 50 mg 2 to 3 times per day.
You may have to monitor blood pressure so that it does not go too low.
<u>Warning:</u> Not to be taken by those with prostate cancer.
~ Ginkgo Biloba 120 mg daily
~ Zeaxanthin 3.75 mg daily
~ Eye Pressure support: Bilberry and Maritime Pine Bark
~ Lutein 10mg daily
~ Coenzyme Q 10 100 to 200 mg daily
Eye Pressure support by Vitaganics (Earl Mindel)
This was a combination of the same ingredients but adding
L-Arginine and Apha Lipoic Acid which I began to take with Dr Bush's protocol. I had taken as many as 900 mg per day of Alpha Lipoic Acid for neuropathy before but was on a maintenance dose of 100 mg/day when I began this regimen.

This foregoing was the protocol that brought my IOP down into the normal range. Others recommended by Life Extension for Glaucoma are listed below. I have taken them sporadically throughout the years and was still taking some but in much smaller dosages.

Vitamin C & Conjunctival Hyperemia
~ Vitamin C 1000 – 2000 mg daily recommended by Life Extension (USA). I was taking much more as listed above and noted a reduction of conjunctival hyperemia exactly as Dr Bush predicted from the very beginning.
~ Acetyl L-Carnitine gradually increasing to 3000 mg per day.

~ Zinc 30 – 50 mg daily
~ Chromium 500 mcg daily
~ Green Coffee 200 – 400 mg daily
~ Green Tea Extract 725 – 1450 mg daily
~ Hydergine's mechanisms may be similar to Forskolii
~ Magnesium 140 -500 mg
I was taking this product in the Cardio Pro which was like Dr Bush's protocol for CardioRetinometry® but I had to add 300 mg more Lysine to match his recommendations.
~ Melatonin 0.3 – 3 mg daily one hour before bed
~ Pyrroloquinoline Quinone 10-20 mg daily
~ Curcumin 400 – 800 mg daily

Reduction of stress must be monitored by all glaucoma patients. Outer stress begets inner stress. Stay away from situations that upset you or people with whom it is difficult to get along. Forgive and forget real or imagined wrongs. Hidden grief may lie in the breast of many of your patients, and it would be worthwhile to ask pertinent questions concerning stressful things in their lives. This could be especially true of age related vision problems where grief could be a causative factor.

Dr Bush was the first to actually measure the effects of stress in the retinal arteriolar plaque as he has often noted. I was impressed when Dr Hedahl confirmed his feelings too about it, i.e., that grief may be part of the problem in glaucoma. This gave me a heads-up to look for further reasons for the sudden and scary diagnosis in my own case.
Below is a list of products that I ordered for glaucoma, in addition to Dr Bush's CardioRetinometry® protocol. Simply stated: This is the program that reduced my IOP.
1~Eye Pressure Support- Life Extension (USA

2~Forskolii -` Life Extension (USA)
3~Super Zeaxanthin - Life Extension (USA)
4~Eye Pressure Support- Vitaganics.

After a good reading of IOP, I stupidly went away to try another company's formulation for Glaucoma. It did not work, but my IOP went even higher at my next visit to my Optometrist. I returned to the original protocol, and my IOP now stands at 18. So far I do not have any additional ONH damage

Due to the ONH damage, I have also added 3 months of Neuroplex, and Neurotrophin Photomorphogen extract from Standard Process, as well as A-C Carbamide, which balances the osmotic pressure in the body. In addition I have made several schedule adjustments to relieve outer stress, and added an Adaptogen before bed to settle myself down, as well as Adrenal support to address the adrenal stress, for which I had been in treatment after the death of my husband.

In addition to all this I added the Mineral Germanium, which at the time, was not approved for humans, only animals. Since that time, I found research where it has been shown to work well for humans in the reduction of IOP, and letting glaucoma patients see again.

Very Personal Experience
Today we are accustomed, almost brainwashed, into demanding double blind placebo controlled, crossover studies before we accept anything. But Sir William Osler would not be recognised as the Father of Modern medicine, and we would have had to wait another 100 years, if we had ignored evidence based medicine.

Potassium cyanide kills. We do not need DBPC studies to prove it. Purists say there is no such thing as a medical proof. If that is true, why do we bother at all with DBPC studies? As the late Dr. Barbara Starfield MD said, the standard of evidence required for the approval of a new drug against the placebo is ridiculously low. Contrast this with the standard of evidence demanded by Medicine for any of the actions of vitamin C, and one sees a huge inconsistency. The discordance of standards is even less acceptable when one considers that part of the approvals process for drugs, is that they be shown to not kill too many people! But nobody can be shown to have died in 80 years of self administration of vitamin C.

The personal history here breaks with tradition. It is necessary. I could not wait to see completion of vitamin C studies that pharmacy and medicine would never fund! Dr. Bush's research work in a US hospital was sabotaged. Forces are at work to prevent people learning and the tradition of not describing one's personal experiences can benefit only the pharmaco-medical industry and business with sickness.

To say such experiences are 'anecdotal,' or 'merely anecdotal,' which is the shibboleth applied to virtually all case studies for vitamin C, but not to other vitamins except vitamin E, is an obstructive device. Indeed Dr Bush's encyclopedia graphs show how, since 1958, medical prejudice against vitamin C has been amply organised and put into effect in the journals. It is irrefutably cast in stone. Anybody can replicate the results of his research in one evening. All that is necessary is to ask the National Library of Medicine search engine (PubMed) to find all the papers mentioning scurvy in each year from the beginning of the database. Repeat the search using the term "Vitamin C AND Deficiency," and one finds that until 1958 there were more mentions of "scurvy" than vitamin C deficiency. After 1958 the graphs simply took off in opposite directions, with vitamin C deficiency hitting the roof and scurvy diving to the bottom. Is it any wonder then that today's physicians scoff and say that scurvy has "gone away!" In the UK they tell patients that "Nobody gets scurvy any more!"

My own very personal history as an experienced health professional is – I therefore suggest – every bit as useful to bear in mind as any huge, but so often badly flawed, double blind placebo controlled study, perhaps carefully designed from the outset to produce the desired result.

Medicine

I know this sounds like a lot, but it is my story and I hope you will look carefully at what you can do to help yourself and your patients with this problem. I had no time to lose, i.e., waiting on results from double blind, placebo controlled studies. My vision was at stake! At my latest appointment, as mentioned before, my Optometrist told me "The way you are going, your eyes are good for another 20 years." Good news for me, within a comparatively short time of the diagnosis.

This same approach with harmless nutrients can be applied to any eye condition. And it is my hope that each student and doctor will relentlessly search for answers for prevention as well as correcting the multitude of eye problems in the US and UK alone, not to mention those conditions in Third World countries. If we wait for the Ophthalmologists whose livings derive from disease, history shows that we might wait another 100 years.

Since Optometrists can tell so much about the human body by what they observe in the eye, I am hoping for more education in this field, as well as a release of restraint, for them to practice what they know. For ten years Optometrists have been encouraged to offer prevention for macular degeneration. We now have a wonderful discovery by Dr Bush where the improvement in vasculature can be measured and observed. He has shown that the arteriolar reflex is predictable in location and reversible, with its disappearance accompanied by widening of the vessels, showing by time-lapse photography, that it was a blockage causing the reflex, not an "ensheathment." Improvement of the vasculature in the eyes is going to benefit not only the heart but the entire system as well. Hypertension might disappear.

May this suppression by medicine become less a pattern as greater efforts are made to reveal the true causes of disease. Could the same thing happen as other new discoveries are made in eye health? Do physicians honestly want prevention? Do they honestly want to promote nutrition? Historically speaking, it seems not. Major General Sir Robert McCarrison (CIE, MA, MD, DSc, LLD, FRCP; 1878 - 1960). was one of the most illustrious doctors of our time. After he returned from the Land of Hunza where disease is almost non-existent, and founded the British Medical Association Nutrition Section, it died with him.

It is tragic that when Dr Bush discovered CardioRetinometry®, he was ignored by Official Medicine and the UK National Health Service for more than a decade, with the General Optical Council discouraging other optometrists from engaging in preventive measures against intraluminal plaque. What a crime against mankind, and for what cause may I ask ? Greed perhaps ? Or protection of one's own turf? Either would be a primitive response, and certainly not for the good of the public!

Concerning the prevention of Age Related Macular Degeneration (ARMD) there is not the opportunity to measure the success as quickly as there is with CardioRetinometry® with the intraluminal plaque. These are three major health concerns with the populace, i.e., heart attacks, strokes and blindness.

Age Related Macular Degeneration (ARMD) occurs, most damagingly, in the foveal region of the human eye, which has a concentration of 2.1 ratio of Zeaxanthin and Lutein, and is the spot where our major vision needs take place. There are also steep vitamin C and vitamin E gradients of retinal concentration radiating outwards from the fovea centralis. The most critical (sharpest) vision is therefore linked to the highest concentration of these two antioxidants. Both atrophic (dry) and neovascular (wet) conditions can take place even simultaneously, and it is a devastating disease, affecting central vision. It is the major cause of blindness in Americans (www.amd.org) The need is to make available to patients, the education and supplementation that will stop this condition from advancing and even to reverse it.

A Nutritionist in every Optometrist's Office?
 When one ingredient is lacking, e.g. Lutein for AMD prevention, one can't eat a bushel of spinach per day no matter how hard one might try.

Supplementation can be offered to make up the deficiency as quickly as possible. Patients can be directed to the correct supplements that are affordable and easily obtainable. In addition to broadening their own knowledge of nutritional needs for good vision, Optometrists in a large group practice might consider employing a Nutritionist, who specializes in Ocular Nutrition able to oversee the inventory specific to vision needs as well as the associated ordering and bookkeeping. Ideally, the prescribing and dispensing should be ongoing as a continuous service that is self funding for patients returning every few months between biennial examinations.

Inevitably, as the fundamental importance of nutrition to both good and prolonged eyesight becomes better appreciated, Optometrists will find themselves sounding more like nutritionists. They have the advantage now clearly revealed, of being able to review and monitor the benefits of that advice in ways not available to Nutritionists without their special training in ocular diagnostics. Clearly we are destined to learn a great deal e.g. about AMD, from each other!

The problem for Optometrists
It is their training and the public expectation which needs raising. We must cultivate enthusiasm in their patients for the new approach. But we must not burden patients with onerous obligations. Buying the simplest foodstuffs has already become a task, e.g., reading the ingredients to avoid the dangerous polyunsaturated oils, so long promoted to us all as healthy! What an untruth! Our bodies never make unsaturated oils. We make saturated fat. Nature knows what is best for us! On the positive side, how

to add to the advice and the list of beneficial, vision preserving nutrients, needs to be carefully considered.

With young people who will 'live forever' and can't imagine ageing, our advice can be a waste of breath. We are also familiar with the 'know it all' types who believe they have little to learn. And then we will continue to suffer those who come from politically minded, or just plainly uninformed physicians with the advice ringing in their ears, "that those Optometrists are "hooked on vitamin C, but "it just "makes expensive urine." It has been observed by those who research cadavers for scientific use, that there is more vitamin C in the eye than anywhere else in the body.

Our reward can only be gained by gentle perseverance and Dr Bush found that the answer to many of these problems of client education in his practice, was to delegate the information giving, to nurses. Patients listen to other staff, particularly reception staff, who need to be well trained to enthuse about the nutrients, particularly vitamin C, and to inform patients how the practice sees major health benefits being gained by those who at least take vitamin C several times a day. Patients quickly learn themselves, when this ameliorates some of their health problems.

Thus, it is not sufficient to tell patients to "take antioxidants" or to "eat lots of fruits and vegetables". Many are doing that already but are still experiencing vision loss or at least lowered levels of Macular Pigment a precursor to ARMD. Practices are not looking for extra costs here, but protecting sight, and caring for people's fears of going blind. The public can only benefit from the two professions working closely together. Of the greatest value is a nutritionist emphasising the need for ascorbate constantly.

The health of the macular pigment is vital to good vision, warding off many eye diseases. Macular degeneration does not have to occur "naturally" as a result of age. We can avoid it through proper nutrition and lifestyle. From Dr Bush's experience, it seems that even risk due to some inherited factors can be reduced, if one abandons family traits by changing diet and lifestyle, so as not to invite this weakness. An example might in time prove to be the avoidance of primary open angle glaucoma when patients adopt the regimen of vitamin C to bowel tolerance.

Dr. Bush's informal finding before he retired from contact lens practice, was that there had been no case of glaucoma or AMD in his patient base for many years amongst those who adopted the vitamin C advice, whereas at least 8 cases were expected. Diabetes also appeared to be in marked decline and coronary thrombosis was non-existent in vitamin C compliant patients. Normally Type II Diabetes is another example where, given the same diet and lifestyle, an entire family line may be affected by this malady, when simple changes would preserve the quality of life, and prevent this degeneration.

Two cases of wet AMD, one referred to Dr. Bush by her physician, and the other a staff nurse, were cured with vision restored. Ordinarily Optometrists would be well advised of the need for anti-angiogenesis drugs to stop or slow the proliferation of blood vessels which can leak and cause additional scarring or further loss of vision. However, it may be the case that vitamins C and E could prove to be better treatments. Eye Surgeons generally agree that photodynamic therapy may halt the condition but is unlikely to improve it The choroidal vessels which carry nutrition to the macula are already in place! We need to cooperate with the system already built into the physio-mechanism to supply the proper nutrition.

As an important preventive measure the CardioRetinometry® program designed by Dr. Bush proves clearing of the retinal vessels in photographic images over a span of more than twelve years since 1998. The major preventive component in his program on which the greatest emphasis was laid during that time and at every contact lens aftercare examination (being at least six monthly) was Vitamin C throughout the entire period. He advised bowel tolerance and dispensed 200 gram pots of sodium L-ascorbate.

The photographic record cannot be denied. It is fact. The food frequency questionnaires became of secondary value. It was obvious from the photographs whether or not the vitamin C was being taken in adequate amounts. Physicians demand more evidence but without imperiling lives and health it is impossible to obtain. The photographs over such a long period of time are proof of an effect.

Physicians can argue and doubt if they wish, that this program does increase the efficacy of all visual needs as well as the entire circulatory system. Patients need little convincing. They have no axe to grind. The very fact that the vessels are cleared by a harmless, non-toxic protocol is sufficient for reasonable people. It opens the pathway for nutritional needs to reach their intended place for repair and maintenance. Physicians say "This is Life Extension."

Orthodox Optometry mandates that with the dry form, which progresses over time, we may supplement; but with wet AMD it may be necessary to treat immediately with drug therapy.

This latter advice may be reviewed as with care, and good and frequent sequential retinal photography, it is now possible to detect incipient wet AMD. Both life style and nutritional adjustments need to be stressed in the general population in order to prevent AMD.

This includes the following:
Do not Smoke!
Protect your eyes from sunlight.
Eat all the dark greens and the brightly colored fruits and vegetables you can.
Take NATURAL vitamin E, 1,000iu/day
And take all the vitamin C you can tolerate!

The dinner plate should reflect a rainbow of colors. Too often meals resemble the mud pies we made as youngsters, with various shades of tan and brown. Think about that for a minute, potatoes, breads, pastas, rice, buns, meats, chicken, pizza. We should have brightly colored greens, reds, yellows, oranges and purples, inviting our appetite to indulge in foods that will not leave us hungry for cookies and cake to finish drowning the meal so it cannot be digested. These brightly colored foods are where the antioxidants are. If that is hard for you to stomach (no pun) then think about how you would feel about going blind later in life? Remember your body will make you answer up for everything you put into it.

Common Diseases of the Eye
I must credit ZeaVision for the following information sent to me, in the process of writing this book. The

POLA Study of *Plasma Lutein and Zeaxanthin and other Carotenoids as Modifiable Risk Factors for Age Related Maculopathy was* done in a Mediterranean population in 1995 and 1997 with 2,584 recruited. It was determined that with supplementation of Lutein and Zeaxanthin, that when the plasma level was high there was a decrease by 75% in the incidence of nuclear cataract.

It was determined that the Zeaxanthin had more beneficial effect than the Lutein.

In another study *Macular Pigment and Visual Performance Under Glare Conditions,* by James M. Stringham, PhD., and Billy R. Hammond. Ph.D., it was determined that supplementation with Lutein and Zeaxanthin, greatly improved the glare tolerance and recovery. This seemed to be commensurate with the increase of Macular Pigment (MP) density.

It is my understanding that anything that will help increase the health of the retina or macula will be advantageous to other conditions as well.
Dry macular degeneration
Wet macular degeneration
Macular holes
Detached retina.

All of those diseases involving the macula need to have certain nutrients to prevent the degeneration.

In his book *Second Spring,* Dr. Maoshing Ni lists 5 secrets to save one's eye sight. These are included in his website and include
(1) Blended juicing,
(2) High antioxidant foods,
(3) Staying hydrated,

4) Eye exercises (not recommended in this book - not dealing with orthoptics) to maintain good vision as well as getting rid if those pesky floaters (Dr Ni), and (5) Instant eye remedies which include Pop- Eye's Tea made daily from Spinach leaves.

He recommends just a few main ingredients that are commonly found so the general public can have access to good vision. It would be important to make sure of the quality (i.e., standardized, organic, etc.) of the ingredients. Some are Grape seed extract, Bilberry and Ginkgo.

Folklore that works for some.

There are many nutrients that increase circulation, not only to the eye but to the ears and brain and the entire head including those that have been studied to aid in the progression of Alzheimers and other forms of dementia, such as Huperzine A, N Acyetyl Cysteine, Alpha Lipoic acid, Quercitin, Japanese Knotweed, Resveratrol, Bacopa. and so forth. All these contain more than vitamins and minerals. We do not know all the phytonutrients and constituents that comprise these plants and minerals. Increasing interest is being shown in neurotransmission and possible ways of reducing cerebral plaque associated with Alzheimer's.

Again we see that good vision includes good health practices with special attention being paid to preserving one's eyesight. Dr Earl Mindell PhD., in his *Vitaganics* supplements has produced a specific formula for reducing eye pressure which includes several of the mentioned ingredients but in smaller quantities. In *The Vitamin Bible* (p145) he lists specific ingredients to address Eye problems. The list includes:
~ Vitamin A - 10,000 units 1-3 times per day for 5 days. Then stop.

~ Time released B 100 complex - AM and PM.
~ Vitamin C 500 mg - with citrus bioflavonoids, rutin, and hesperidin - one AM and one PM. (Edits author)
~ Vitamin E - 500 units AM and PM.
The vitamin C content in this formula is of course in addition to the mega doses (12 to up to 100 grams) given as sodium ascorbate as prescribed by Pauling and Bush.

The fact that Dr. Rimm found that 1 gram of vitamin C had a barely measurable effect on IOP (noted also by Virno et. al.) may be accounted for by the time scale. One gram of vitamin C would act to reduce IOP by slow renovation of the trabeculum, whereas Virno et al followed by Prof. Bietti, in the Rome University Eye Clinic, were intent on using the osmolarity of daily 30 gram doses in four x 7.5 gram intakes.

Adelle Davis again advises anti stress nutrition composed of whole foods to bring the health of the body up to par. Stress is thought to be a causative factor in Glaucoma as well as other disease conditions in the body.

I must emphasise that we can wait forever for double blind placebo controlled studies and considering the risk to benefit ratio – on balance it is best for health professionals to voice their informal opinions. Without evidence based medicine we would still be in the 19th Century.

Exactly as predicted by our teaching, after my own husband passed away, as is so commonly found, I experienced the same adrenal problems and upset circadian rhythms. as is the case with so many widows and widowers. After that was almost brought into balance, I had three accidents and then I was diagnosed with the open angle glaucoma.

In any trauma or stress the body's demand for certain nutrients can be depleted, and in the case of vitamin C, beyond one's ability to meet the extra demands without mega supplementation.

Vitamin B and Psychiatry
What next? The B vitamins which are not stored in the body may be less problematical for most but in some psychiatric conditions, it has been found that Niacin particularly may need mega supplementation as niacinamide. Dr. Abram Hoffer and Dr Humphrey Osmond* may have been the first to discover this. Interestingly, all these can be linked to the fifty odd factors in Dr Bush's encyclopedia that precipitate scurvy related diseases because of increased and unmet vitamin C needs. (* See references at chapter end)

Discerning
Davis goes on to say, In addition, that salt is lost in this condition and the ageing eye with its less elastic tissue (due to cross-linking) does not drain the fluids as it once did thereby increasing intraocular pressure which can eventually lead to Optic Nerve Head (ONH) damage and resulting blindness if not treated in time.
Bietti concluded in 1966, at the time Adelle Davis was writing her book, that collapse of the collagen in the trabeculum, could be the cause of POAG when he noted that reduction of IOP persisted after cessation of the 30 grams of oral vitamin C his cohort had consumed every day in four doses of 7.5 grams.

She had seen the anti-stress diet, clear up glaucoma when taken 6 times per day, as long as the patient continues with the higher salt diet. Though every case is specific to the individual, adding salt to the diet so the adrenals can produce cortisone is imperative. In addition sodium ascorbate with its small salt content can make up for salt deficiency while helping not only the eye, but the entire cardio vascular system

Because it is so very important for Optometrists to bear in mind, I repeat that, as noted in Dr Bush's *700 Vitamin C Secrets* (page 240-242, #783-788) we find a references to Bietti, 1966, even to the repair of the spongy trabeculum, which in turn allows proper drainage through the Canal of Schlemm, and consequent reduction of the intraocular pressure.

Collagen again
How many Optometrists would ever have imagined that Primary Open Angle Glaucoma might be a 'collagen' or 'scorbutic' disease raising IOP and the vascular component compounding the felony by driving the ischaemia of the Optic Nerve head? Could this explain the bizarre results obtained with G.. Timolol? C.f. the appendicectomy case that dies post operatively after a successful procedure because of complications from the antibiotics?

Appendicitis; arterial disease, connected?
Could both the appendicitis, and the subsequent post-operative infections, share the same aetiology, and be one more example, like the coronary artery bypass, of surgery being employed to treat a deficiency disease? How many Optometrists can now admit that at this point, they have not made the connection, and started in their own minds reviewing their opinions about the merits of iridencleisis and trabeculectomy?

I will add that with glaucoma, keeping the stress level under control is extremely important and now we know why, if we accept the foregoing. The patient must always be careful to obtain adequate diet according to the amount of stress.

Without the proper salt content in our diets the adrenals cannot make the Cortisol and the entire ability of the body to handle stress is disrupted, often resulting in high IOP, and a multitude of other biological malfunctions. So the dreaded sodium, banned from our diets by our physicians, might head us into even greater trouble.

Davis addresses unrelenting negative emotions as being an underlying cause of stress. With this in mind, as for many physical ailments, it behooves us to forgive and forget trespasses against us. To hold ill feelings, only hurts the one holding them. My Mother. Ruth Branch Merrill, a Qualified Nutritionist, used to say "To hold a grudge against another only puts poison into your own body. " I can hear her say so, as if it were only yesterday.

I also have found with Life Extension (USA) that the addition of high doses of Bilberry will act to decrease IOP as well as Forskolii and Zeaxanthin. These two antioxidants are found in a 2.1 ratio in the fovea (the yellow spot) which is a major player in our vision process. A deficiency would result in thinning of the macular pigment and consequent degeneration which leads to blindness.

In another study done by Dr Kazuhiko Asai, PhD, who dedicated his life to the study of Germanium, he discovered many eye diseases are helped by this mineral. Germanium alone has decreased IOP and restored vision in glaucoma patients so they cry out "I can see!" Quoting from the Regenerative Nutrition Website www.regenerativenutrition.org

"I am sometimes reminded of the blind patients who often came to my office. There were diseases of the retinal blood vessels, such as glaucoma, black cataracts, detached retinas, inflammation of the retina and optic nerves, and without exaggeration, I can say that it was amazing how effective germanium had been. I often witnessed scenes where patients wept as they cried out, 'Now I can see.' Those who could not see would invariably say, 'If I could only see again, Doctor, I would give anything. If it were money I would even go into debt to pay for it.' I cannot understand the psychology of people who know the joy of seeing, and yet do evil things and are greedy. There can be no greater happiness in the world than being able to see. During the International Angiological Congress, I met a professor of Ophthalmology at the State Medical College of Rio de Janeiro. He wrote that "using the germanium compound on a patient virtually blind with amaurosis yielded amazingly good results, and that the patient was well on the road to recovery." It had already been verified that germanium rejuvenates retinal vessels, and is therefore effective in treating glaucoma and amaurosis. His letter has added new evidence of its efficacy.

Detached retina, in some cases nutritional? It is thought to be from a lack of Vitamin E or C. Davis recommends the addition of Vitamin E, 150 iu's, to babies, but my question is the ability of the liver to handle fats in an infant at this early age unless given as an emulsion or to the nursing mother who can supply it in lactation to the nursing infant. See below

Dr. Bush's encyclopedia 700 Vitamin C Secrets (1526, 1527)

Retinitis, too can have many causes. Today we would think of high dose vitamin C while noting that it is corrected by a high protein diet in addition to complete nutrition. Care should be noted if the patient is not digesting and absorbing protein and correction should be made by digestive enzymes and or Betaine Hydrochloride (HCL. Davis).

Here it might be best to quote Dr. Bush's encyclopedia.

1526. Retinal Detachment: Retinal detachment: where due to vitreoretinal traction and peripheral tearing spontaneously resolving or curable caught early. Assessment for laser prophylaxis is desirable in every case without exception. This is when an ophthalmologist can be worth his weight in gold. Serous retinopathy and, of course, macular holes are a risk.

1527. Retinal detachment and tortuosity: Where due to vessel tortuosity caused by atherosclerosis leading to blockage of arteriolar flow or venous return, intraretinal stress lines precede the retinal tear with subsequent detachment, the complete aetiology being revealed by sequential retinal images, also showing how it is predictable. The prevention of the tortuosity would have avoided and prevented the traction, then the tearing and detachment. Sudden irreversible blindness due to thrombosis of the central artery or vein of the retina is a concomitant risk until the atherolysis shows reduction of the atheroma. The thrombosis supports the author's opinion that the arteriolar reflex derives in fact much more from intraluminal plaque, itself the origin of the thrombus.

Cataracts

Much research has been done to determine the cause of cataracts. They can be produced in animals of all kinds by withdrawing Vit B2 from the diet. Also human babies who cannot tolerate galactose (a milk sugar) can develop cataracts. When B2 is added to the diet of animals and people alike the cataracts disappear. In animals deficient of Pantothenic acid, when given this supplement, the cataracts will disappear.

Massive doses of Vitamin C will clear up drug induced cataracts by clearing the body of the drugs. These are often in weight loss drugs. In addition, increasing the circulation to the eye is paramount to carry these valuable vision nutrients to the eyes. Again, exercises to increase circulation to the eyes are important.

Stress is a major factor in developing cataracts especially if it is prolonged, and is also the case with the development of glaucoma. The importance of stress management is something of which we should all be more aware because stress is an underlying cause of much ill health and especially so with those who have cataracts or glaucoma. These two nutrients B2 and Pantothenic acid are necessary for the production of cortisone.

Please be guided by your doctor if you are supplementing B Vitamins. In both cases, complete nutrition, Vitamin C and E, as well as sufficient protein must be followed for complete recovery. Here again, a regimen that includes complete nutrition, as recommended by Adelle Davis as well as other nutritionists, is excellent to avoid over supplementation.

Some conditions do require mega doses as prescribed by your health care provider, but one should not rely on self diagnosis and prescription, without the guidance of a professional. However in the case of Vitamin C your bowel tolerance is your dose limit. With H_2O_2 it is the nausea that determines your dose limit as you work toward your maximum limit
Selenium

A selenite type of cataract is possible and has been noted. This is one of the mineral supplements that must be approached with caution. The recommended amount is usually estimated to lie between 50 and 100 micrograms/day. Perplexingly, it displays cataractogenic and anti-cataract properties. The work of Dawczynski J, Winnefeld K, et.al. is noteworthy. [Selenium and cataract--risk factor or useful dietary supplement?]. Klin Monbl Augenheilkd. 2006 Aug;223(8):675-80.

Choroiditis; See retinitis.
Curcumin.
A yellow herb much favored in India, otherwise known as Turmeric, with pronounced Anticataractogenic properties. See Manikandan R, Thiagarajan R, et al. Curcumin prevents free radical-mediated cataractogenesis through modulations in lens calcium.Free Radic Biol Med. 2010 Feb 15;48(4):483-92. Epub 2009 Dec 10.
A warning is given here by Dr Bush in limiting B2 to 2 mg per day in supplements. There is a possibility that a mega dose might cause detachment of the retina due
to vitreal liquefaction. It is described in Appendix 3.
Blurred vision. (and conjunctival hyperemia) Paralysis of the muscles behind the eyes is corrected by B vitamins, particularly B 1, (Davis). Blurred vision may

also be due to viscous tears resulting, particularly, from an allergic reaction in the palpebral and bulbar conjunctiva. The antihistaminic action of ascorbate may dispel it. It can also be cleared by taking an infusion of Celandine Tea. (Dr. Shook, *Advanced Herbology*, p.288) A stronger decoction is also listed in that book but an infusion may be all that is necessary for our purposes.

Corneal abnormalities

See Dr Bush's *700 Vitamin C Secrets* page 191, 192 # 469-471, for Corneal conditions and the use of Vitamin C eye drops and intravenous applications. CardioRetinometry® is again referred to as the window to the heart.

Protruding Eye (Proptosis)

The common cause is toxic thyroid as in hyperthyroidism.

Treating the thyroid deficiency is necessary for long term results. This is accomplished by thyroid nourishment, iodine supplementation and stress reduction. A Nutritionist should oversee this condition.

In hypothyroid, many T4 and T3 tests taken from serum do not show the deficiency. A simple patch lest on the inner wrist will suffice to show if the thyroid is low. If the Iodine patch disappears before 24 hours there is a deficiency that does not show up in blood tests. Many women who are overweight are told by their doctors that their thyroid is okay when in fact it is not. It may not have developed enough to cause this manifestation in the eye but it shows in their inability to lose weight.

Another condition causing a protruding eye is an auto-immune disease, which should be medically monitored. It usually causes hyperthyroid and can be treated with homeopathic remedies as well. There are also available homeopathic remedies to ameliorate this condition. Some drugs for facial acne also cause thyroid cancer and resulting protruding eyes. Optometrists are expected to be knowledgeable about the possibility of these conditions when treating patients and refer them to the proper doctors.

If you memorize this your patients will thank you, a plethora of eye problems come up in regular eye exams that have very simple solutions nutritionally. Quoting from Adelle Davis *Let's Get Well*, page 281, on Vitamin A and vision:

"Visual problems associated with a mild lack of Vitamin A include premature tiring of the eyes, sensitivity to bright lights and glare, dimness of vision at night, (a common cause of car accidents) less acute day vision, and susceptibility to such infections as styes, conjunctivitis, iritis, and corneal ulcers." Less than 5,000 units per day can result in other conditions such as Bitot's spots, which reverses quickly in taking 50,000 units of Vitamin "A" daily. Vitamin C helps.

Retinitis: Many causes. Evaluation of high dose ascorbate by sequential fundus photography gives the opportunity to reveal a cause or a cure. Referral to ophthalmologist for second opinion always.

Retinitis pigmentosa: It is less likely that the optometrist will be the first to detect this condition, usually spotted early in life. It is another condition that if left unchecked, will result in blindness. In addition to complete nutrition there are now available, antioxidant supplements that increase macular pigment so that it does not have to continue its downward trend toward blindness caused by the Bassen-Kornzweig syndrome and prevented by massive doses of vitamins A, E and presumably C. Pauling "How To Live Longer and Feel Better," p.280.)

There are in addition nine or ten different types of retinal involvement which are reversed by nutrition and CardioRetinometry. (700 Vitamin C Secrets, Dr Bush, p 362, 363 Numbers 1525 – 1536.)

Uveitis: Feared most is Acute Anterior Uveitis in the treatment of which Optometrists are very well trained Avoidance of complications calls for urgent and every possible treatment. Obviously, liposomal vitamin C whilst dispatching the patient to hospital. Cathcart states that it is curable with 30,000 to 100,000mgs of ascorbic acid in 4 to 15 doses every 24 hrs.

Vitamin B deficiencies have a long list of common eye conditions that are often ignored until a serious condition arises. Whenever asthenopia has been eliminated by prescribed lenses, the Optometrist might consider other causes of "blood shot eyes . . . pain on exposure to bright lights . . . cracked outer eye corners,. . . burning eyes. . . red eyes . . . watering. . . itching . . . sandy eyelids . . . intolerance to light . . . abnormally dilated pupils . . . blurred and dim vision . . increased winking of the eyelids . . . inability to see under poor illumination . . . inability to focus sharply . . . eye strain after close work." Most of the burning and gritty feelings may be due to histamine. Vitamin C in sufficient amounts was found in Dr Bush's practice to greatly reduce contact lens wearing discomfort. He could not get it published in Optometry journals beholden to the pharmacy.

(See the well kept secret of the metabolic conversion of histamine to hydantoin-5-acetic acid.)

Less common symptoms include "disturbances in recognizing colors, objects and people" as well as other abnormalities.

Since Vitamin C and the B Vitamins are not stored in the body it is necessary for us to be aware of these symptoms that are signaling to the patient that the body needs help. If Optometrists can recognize these insufficiencies then many serious eye diseases can be eliminated before they develop into full blown cases resulting in blindness or other conditions that are untreatable. What a wonderful thing to be a part of the solution against blindness

Dr Jonathan Wright says that it is necessary to add zinc to the diet when adding Vitamin A for night vision.   (P 315 *Nutritional Healing*) Improvement occurs about 3 months after supplementation and increases as the dose is continued. However, care must be taken that a copper deficiency does not occur in long term zinc supplementation.

Emotional blindness:
Different from the sudden blindness of homonymous hemianopia of migraine that can be suffered whilst driving. Situations that can no longer be tolerated by an individual can also cause blindness.

As a young girl, I was acquainted with a woman who was blind. She told me that she became blind when she saw a brick wall collapse, killing her young husband. It happened in England she said. After that she could not see and came back to America living out her life as a blind widow. Her house was sparsely furnished and her clothing was gray and colorless as was her home.

Optometrists who specialize in contact lens fitting will be wondering when I am going to deal with hay fever. It is a non-event when people find the right amount of sodium ascorbate that suits them! The histamine is converted into harmless CO_2 and H_2O. Dr Bush says all the 'wet' lens research was unnecessary.

* References:
Irvine DG. Apparently non-indolic Erhlich-positive substances related to mental illness.
J Neuropsychiatr.1961 Aug;2:292-305.

Hoffer A. The presence of malvaria in some mentally retarded children. ArnlMentDef:
1963:67:730-732.
Iwine DG. Kryptopyrrole in molecular psychiatry. In: Hawkins D, Pauling L, eds.

Orthomolecular Psychiatry: Treatment of Schizophrenia. San Francisco: WH Freeman and Company: 1973:146-178.
Hoffer A. The discovery of kryptopyrrole and its importance in diagnosis of biochemical
imbalances in schizophrenia and in criminal behavior. J Orthomolec Med. 1995 First Quarter:10:3-7.

================

Footnote:
This is not available on PubMed because nutrition and vitamin cures are suppressed by the NIH/ National Library of Medicine. Google finds the research.

Canal of Schlemm
It had always been thought that blockage of the Canal of Schlemm was a principal contributory factor in the

rise of intraocular pressure. Bush considers that the seminal work of Virno et al repeated and confirmed by Bietti, in the Rome University Eye Clinic, following the successful lowering of IOP was due to recover of the hypothesised collapsed trabeculum. This may have been accompanied by recovery of the Canal of Schlemm.

In this chapter I have been at pains to emphasise the need for us to learn from ourselves. Our own personal experiences teach us best of all what we cannot expect to live long enough for medical science to discover and confirm, to teach us.

Chapter IV
Vitamin C: The Master Nutrient and CardioRetinometry®

Used by permission of Sydney Bush, DOpt,.

 Primarily we expect that CardioRetinometry® will serve throughout a lifetime to inform – as we age – regarding our growing dependence on dietary ascorbate as our latter years draw nearer. We can only guess that lack of the L-gulono-lactone-gamma oxygen 2-oxidoreductase, gene, the enzyme that catalyzes the terminal step of L-ascorbic acid biosynthesis in mammalian liver, was meant to be unexpressed for good reasons. May et al., have shown to a degree, how in some ways our red cells give us an advantage over animals that convert their blood glucose to ascorbate! For me, the burning questions are –

1.   What if our gene were to be restored?
2.   How do the mysterious fraction of people who continue to excrete vitamin C whilst on an exclusion diet, make it?
3. Why, when these people were occasionally revealed in medical studies, were they never investigated?
POLITICS!
We wait for many answers. Such has been the prejudice that most of the research along the lines indicated by Dr. Frederick R Klenner MD has been deliberately avoided. Only one trial of ten gram doses has been carried out. That was in the UK by Dr. Kale Kenton. But it was never published. We wonder why.
 Throughout his life, the scientist who brought the

World's attention to the subject – Dr. Linus Pauling with 90 PhDs – was unable to get more than two papers published in peer reviewed medical journals recognised and reported by the National Library of Medicine. People have repeatedly assured me that my work will not be recognised until I study for a PhD instead of being satisfied with a PhD Honoris Causae of little known and unaccredited Cosmopolitan University. I point to the most distinguished scientist of the 20th Century and ask them if they seriously believe any more PhDs would have made a jot of difference after 70 years of medical stone walling. Official Medicine even refuses to recognise the (honest) Journal of Orthomolecular Medicine, and to consider the appeals of expert committees against a "genocidal" RDA for vitamin C!

MORE FACTS: Dr. Pauling had, before his death at over 92, amassed a PhD for virtually every year of his life! I doubt his record of 90 PhDs will ever be exceeded. Only one man might succeed. That is Pauling's friend Prof. Denham Harman MD., PhD., Father of the Free Radical Theory of Aging and Disease (Nov 1954.) He is still waiting for his Nobel Prize.

He made the most outstanding contribution to public health of the 20th Century unless you think Pauling just wins. But he won't get the Nobel Prize even posthumously, because it would damage medical and pharmacy profits. They go to vast expense and trouble to avoid stimulating interest in antioxidants in general, and vitamin C in particular.

So with 90 PhDs, Official Medicine was so determined to keep him out of the medical archive that, disgracefully, one of the greatest scientists had to pay to have a paper published in Medical Hypotheses and only reluctantly, did the National Academy of Science, of which he was a member, agree to publish his first paper. I am therefore not prepared to waste my life as they want me to, like Don Quixote tilting at windmills, punching the medical tide, submitting useless research proposals to await their pleasure of further rejections. It all delays my objective of publication on PubMed somehow, papers to educate the public and resistant University professors who are opposed to Pauling-Rath theory of arterial disease.

Cosmopolitan University
This is one of the very few Universities believed to not be beholden to funding by pharmaceutical companies. It willingly helped and was the first to create a Faculty of Optometry and CardioRetinometry®. Cosmopolitan University is honest. For many of the others they were not allowed to support any efforts that may infringe on the financial interests of their funding sources. Optometry journals have also been reduced in their influence in eye health due to the funding source requirements. And certainly they would not be accepting articles, studies or abstracts on cardiovascular research if that infringed on their financial interests. We need to go beyond these miniscule blockages in the advancement of health and continue to disseminate information as we see new evidences surface.
..Too much of health care is based on the premise of creating a sick society that can be treated with only the drugs provided by the pharmaceutical companies. (Dr Erickson's own medical doctor says "We do not have a health care system but a sick care system in this nation." Further - "No one pays until you get sick.")

157

My NHS contract was threatened if I did not stop advising patients of the hope of preventing or reversing cardio vascular events.

Hull University Department of Engineering is entitled to respect for their rare honesty. They helpfully seconded a BSc student who gained first class honours for a thesis on CardioRetinometry® (Analysis of Retinal Images for Health Care) It is hoped that the Faculty of Medicine will be as open minded as possible and not bring pressure to bear through a threat to the university's funding. That is a worrying possibility. Thank you Mr Gavin Cutler and Dr J. M. Gilbert.

Medical Teaching

Earlier I challenged the Professor of Physiology at Hull-York Medical School, asking him regarding his syllabus, what is being taught, and learned that there is nothing being taught regarding vitamin C and either Hypercholesterolemia, Diabetes, or Allergy. Would CardioRetinometry® be welcome? I do not intend wasting my life on a useless PhD degree guaranteeing nothing; that can – in any case - be granted or withheld on a whim, as happened to well known nutritionist, Patrick Holford. Linus Pauling had 90 PhD's and could not get into the peer reviewed medical journals.   Medical obstruction begins by insisting on PhDs! It is so shameful on graduation day, to see the empty heads of the newly qualified physicians, denied key facts.

Physiology

Vitamin C is so powerful because each molecule contains two readily available free electrons that can be donated to quench a cascade of free radicals. Our cells are full of molecules of all types and varieties, like the ladies at a dance. Imagine a hundred couples twirling round a ballroom and a man collapses, dies, and is removed. Without a partner, she grabs any passing man. The second, now unaccompanied woman becomes a free radical and grabs the nearest man, setting off a chain reaction as every dispossessed woman immediately grabs the nearest man who does not belong to her. The presence of one or two well behaved gentlemen, around the dance floor, waiting patiently for partners, represent extra antioxidants, ready to quench trouble immediately when it arises. So the presence of the surplus male partners, calms and stabilizes the event with all the ladies confidently knowing that trouble cannot arise due to the presence of a pool of available gentlemen. It is insurance.

Thus stability is achieved throughout all one's molecules and our genetic makeup is protected from damage. The mitochondrial DNA is protected by extra antioxidants because of the oxidizing chemical reactions within cells that perform phagocytosis, dissolving pathogenic viruses and bacteria.

Phagocytosis and respiratory burst:
It is perhaps over simplifying it if I say that this is the special way in which vitamin C develops free radicals within the cytoplasm of the polymorphonuclear cells, and simultaneously protects the cell from them with myeloperoxidase whilst it forms superoxide, hydrogen peroxide and hypochlorous acid to kill the pathogen. So without vitamin C the phagocytes have neither bullets nor internal defensive armour. The hypochlorous acid is fifty times more bactericidal than the hydrogen peroxide. Bolscher, B.G.J.M. et al."*Vitamin C stimulates the chlorinating activity of human myeloperoxidase [Ascorbic acid]."* Biochim-Biophys-Acta-Protein-Struct-Mol-Enzymol.
Amsterdam : Elsevier Biomedical Press. Jan 31, 1984. v. 784 (2/3) p. 189-191

Phagocytosis and superoxide.

Ascorbic acid neutralises excessive levels of reactive oxidants produced during the action of phagocytes during chronic infection. Ascorbic acid deficiency changes the characteristics of the phagocytic cells and the amount of antibacterial complement contained in the cytoplasm which is needed to greatly enhance the killing and defensive power of the phagocyte. There is a very tight relationship between the amount of vitamin C available in the blood stream and the effectivity of the phagocytes. (Anderson R. Lukey P.T. A biological role for ascorbate in the selective neutralisation of extracellular phagocyte-derived oxidants. Ann. N.Y. Acad. Sci. 1987: 498: 229-247.) Dramatically shown in the catfish, they all died without the vitamin C and all recovered against the bacterial infection with the vitamin C. Li Y, & Lovell RT. "Elevated levels of dietary ascorbic acid increase immune responses in channel catfish." J Nutr. 1985 Jan;115(1):123-31.

Re-reduction of dehydroascorbate:

May et al have demonstrated using 14C-labeled ascorbate and dehydroascorbate, that the oxidised (lost electrons) form of the vitamin C which had been thought to be of no further use in humans, is selectively taken up by the glucose transporter - GLUT – at a rate 10 times faster than that for ascorbate. Then, May's team found that this oxidised vitamin C in the red cells is magically converted back into active reducing ascorbate! Then the team went on to show that the mechanism is so efficient, that they calculated the ability of the red cells to convert the entire oxidised vitamin C in the bloodstream back into potently free radical quenching vitamin C every three minutes! Astonishingly, few researchers appear to know this.

As previously mentioned, one would reasonably have expected a fanfare of publicity for the discovery of this amazing and important mechanism, no matter how embarrassing to Official Medicine! May, Qu and the confusingly named - for a haematologist - Dr. Whitesell - did really brilliant work! May J.M, Qu Z, Whitesell R.R, *Ascorbic acid recycling enhances the antioxidant reserve of human erythrocytes.* Biochemistry 1995. 34:12721-12728.

Offers to the British Medical Journal and the Journal of Medical Ethics of letters or papers on scurvy, resulted in rejection of any possibility of publication. Statins: It is also hoped that the light will dawn soon re the damaging effects of the cholesterol hypothesis put forth as actual fact without clinical or laboratory proof of the cardio vascular health of the public.

Marketed as life promoting they have never, since their introduction in the 1980s, achieved life extension. One can imagine the fanfare of publicity during the past 25 years if they had! In the USA users of the Lifestream® cholesterol monitor quickly found that vitamin C was better than statins and with no risk of fatal or damaging side effects.

The Japanese have used Natto for a very long time to balance blood cholesterol which has no damaging effects to the liver. Besides that the proof that, that is an issue with cardio-vascular health is yet to be demonstrated.

Disgraceful omissions in UK National Health Service
In the UK, our National Health Service ambulances are still empty of vitamin C filled hypodermic syringes. They are the immediate antidote to carbon monoxide

poisoning and people die because they are not given the 'flash oxidiser' that Klenner found so effective. Nor are victims of anaphylactic shock given the antihistamine vitamin C injection that neutralises every toxin of every snake, every toxin of every insect, and all heavy metal poisoning. Nor can people who have suffered stroke expect to be recovering immediately in their ambulance but will be further damaged instead by reperfusion injury because of medical intransigence.

After reading this one cannot be surprised that the UK National Health Service withdrew my contract! I refused to promise to stop informing everyone that arterial disease is reversible! Instead – I have 200 written testimonials from delighted patients who agreed, having witnessed their own arterial rejuvenation.

Britain is therefore probably the most medically corrupt country in the world. I learned that a foreign doctor had said "This is a dangerous country in which to be sick!"

Mnemonic:
Outside a red cell, one vitamin C molecule said to another. "I think I've lost an electron"
The second vitamin C Molecule says – "Are you sure?"
First vitamin C molecule replies. "Yes. I am positive!"

This section contains general guidelines for good health, as well as a complete list of the supplements recommended by Dr Sydney Bush in his CardioRetinometry® Program. It is probably the most valuable collection of health information available for your insurance against cardiac arrest, strokes, aneurysms and many other ill health conditions that are becoming more and more "diseases of the young," not just the aged. Just call to mind the news reports you hear in any given year of young, fit, strong, physically active sports persons who "suddenly" die of a heart attack while performing at their top level of expertise and skill in any spectator sport.

The foundation was laid long before. It was not "sudden." Gradually, over years, the cardio- vascular system was compromised bringing about the so called "sudden" failure when it could have been avoided by these health practices. Please take this information seriously. Your life depends on it.

Now Dr. Bush's CardioRetinometry® shows the preventable risk to our lives that everybody had seen but nobody had understood before!

~~~~~~

Nutritional Preventive CardioRetinometry® Males age 30-60 yrs.
Standard Diet and Supplementation Sheets (The Bush view.)

This is the standard advice and Rx for CardioRetinometry® registrants age 30-60yrs (the average age of registrants) who have 'average' health and medical history.

60% of men die of coronary thrombosis or a related episode –e.g. aneurysm or stroke, and that is the fate that awaits the person with 'average' arterial disease. Consider that if 60% of people die of coronary thrombosis or stroke, and many have died of cancer, who would have died of coronary thrombosis, 60% as a figure underestimates the scale of the problem.

"Everything in moderation"

simply does not work! Average arteries = average blood pressure = average age = average thrombosis risk = average heart attack. Prevention of each of these is now possible but ultimately we will still die of a cardiovascular event; cancer, avoidable/curable infection (neglect or medical malpractice) or dementia, or the heart simply falters and stops possibly due to its failure to produce enough Co-Enzyme Q10 which may be what kills many on STATINS! (No Inquests!)

Other causes of death: Dangers of Toximolecular medication

106,000 die annually in US hospitals given properly prescribed medications with 1,000,000 injured annually. (UK and the rest of the West almost certainly in proportion.) (Lazarou, Pomeranz, JAMA. Incidence of adverse drug reactions in hospitalized patients: a meta-analysis of prospective studies. 1998 Apr 15; 279(15):1200-5.)

Risk of death or injury due to supplements

The US centre for control in 2008 found not a single case of death, injury or self harm due to use of supplements bought from health sources and used as directed. Vitamin C's laxative effect is often quoted by doctors as a 'problem.' The only isolated cases of injury were caused by doctors misusing them.

Risk reduction:

Starts immediately with the first dose of vitamin C! It increases with any of over 50 factors that challenge plasma vitamin C status. (See Pp 232-233 of the encyclopaedia - "700 Vitamin C Secrets and 1,000 not so secret for Doctors!")

BEST DIET: SUMMARY: ATKINS DIET WITH GREENS AND SUPPLEMENTS.

Least carbohydrates. Supplemented sensibly with vitamins and nutrients. No Cereals.

Cereals also cause osteoporosis worsened by skimmed milk (no sat fat to absorb Vit D3 and cereal locks up the calcium as phytate) avoid excess saturated fat but we make it!

Meat Fish, eggs, milk, cheeses, all without restriction except pork and lard due to POLYUNSATURATED OILS (PUFAs) in pig feed. EAT AS MANY EGGS AS YOU LIKE. THEY ARE EXCELLENT FOOD FOR THE RETINA AND CANNOT HARM THE HEART AS YOU WILL SEE. You soon tire of excess eggs.

Least fried and cooked under 100 Centigrade. Lightly fried omelettes but it is a pity to fry tomatoes. They should be eaten raw and one/day is a very good rule. Always have extra vitamin C after preserved meats of all kinds to neutralise the nitrosamines (cancer) All bakery products are suspect. Be vigilant: If they say "MADE WITH BUTTER" in big letters, look for PUFAs included in the small print! It started in Spain with every one of the Spanish Omelettes in the supermarkets now with rapeseed or 'vegetable' oil PUFAs.

But they have "Artesanos – potato crisps fried in Olive Oil! Be warned. They are so exceptionally tasty that they become very dangerous to the waistline.

GENERAL:

Polyunsaturated oils (PUFAs) MUST be reduced to an absolute minimum as they increase the need for antioxidants and may cause type 2 diabetes. Omega 3 oils are polyunsaturated but are measured in capsules kept in the dark. Bottled cod liver oil is ill advised due to oxidation even if kept in the dark in the fridge. ONLY Capsules are advised and not after use by date.

Culinary PUFAs are probably causing immense ill health and fish and chip shops should be banned from using them. Vegetarians refusing beef dripping and insisting on bad rape seed type oil are probably contributing to widespread cancer

Note: The half life of plasma vitamin C above the renal threshold is 30 minutes. Below that the person's allele type has a hugely variable effect on survivability.

BEST OILS & FATS

Coconut
Palm (unrefined)
Olive (Virgin)
Butter (NEVER SPREADABLE!
Leave enough for 3 days out of the fridge)
Beef dripping, mutton fat.
Goose /chicken fat.

WORST OILS
Refined Sunflower, Safflower, Rapeseed, Corn, Groundnut. These create vitamin E debt in brain, nerves, cardiovascular and our antioxidant systems.

SUPPLEMENTARY OILS:
Must be before use by date. Always in capsules kept in the dark.

BEVERAGES
Cellular water is far the best. Hull, England, tapwater is excellent with vitamin C (or boiled) to eliminate the chlorine.

PUB: (Public house)
Offer £1 for a pint of tap water with ice, add a little vitamin C and you will outlive the rest. They will make more profit than on beer?
Red wine for its Resveratrol.
Chinese green tea without doubt. Milk may not be so damaging to the polyphenols as thought.

Chinese green tea ground to powder in a few *seconds* in a coffee mill makes VERY strong instant tea that doesn't block the kitchen sink. Very medicinal. Make it in a cafetiere? Drink it light green not dark.

Weak instant coffee and ordinary tea. No problems. Strong instant coffee (more than a level spoon?) may be too much.

Organic coffee beans supposed to be very healthful.

WHOLE MILK.

ORGANIC. Excellent.

Women may be giving themselves osteoporosis drinking skimmed milk!

Hypnotised by the hype that it contains more calcium! Pity. Without the fat it cannot be absorbed. WORSE! Nor can the vitamin D be absorbed that is needed for strong bones as every baby knows, to avoid rickets.

MILK and CEREALS: Osteoporosis risk! The calcium in the milk is locked up by the Phytic acid in the cereals so if you have skimmed milk, the calcium is all wasted and – even if you have WHOLE milk – there may not be enough calcium left to be taken into the body with the milk fat!

ORGANIC whole milk? May be best for younger men to avoid 'moobs,' which may be a risk of the hormones in milk. Need older men worry? Yes!

Best meat. Grass fed of course. Butchers who proudly advertise 'barley fed beef' are doing us no favours. Meat every day for men especially is a good philosophy but it tends to be fattening if carbs are included.

SWEETENERS

Sugar (breaking down to glucose and fructose) blocks the entry of vitamin C and insulin into cells. The fructose it produces causes obesity and addiction. Demerara or any other is still sugar. Yudkin describes it as "sweet, white, and deadly." It raises blood cholesterol but that is NOT the cause of arterial disease. Its glucose blocks the vitamin C portals into cells which causes cholesterol to be needed for physical strengthening as collagen is weakened. CRet plans include collagen support for under 30s but excess glucose frustrates all attempts to penetrate into cells. Lipospheric vitamin C, able to penetrate and support cells freely, overcomes that problem but at the considerable cost of perhaps 4 sachets / day costing 70pence each - over £1,000yr at current prices without considering other nutrients. The strength of the vitamin in the blood stream falls by 50% every 30 minutes to renal threshold. [Glucose–Ascorbate antagonism theory (Ely)]

ARTIFICIAL SWEETENERS:
Saccharin is almost certainly safe and can be used without restriction. Some acidity is claimed but may be exaggerated .
Herbal sweeteners as used in organic supplements are safe.
Cyclamate with caution. Spanish Gov't says it is safe after banning it.

ASPARTAME is POISON
(Canderelle, Equal, Nutrasweet etc. Very dangerous.)
Aspartame breaks down to
1. Formic acid (Ant sting poison)
2. Formaldehyde (Embalming fluid, disinfectant)
3. Methyl alcohol. (Wood spirit) Blinds people.

SOFT DRINKS:
Home made is best, with sodium ascorbate powder poured in after dissolving in a glass water jug, lemon juice or a Lidl bottle of lemon juice. Next best may be Hermesetas or other saccharin, and pop in a couple of Lidl effervescent 1 gram tablets of vitamin C to gas up

the bottle* (A lemonade type pressure bottle of course!" Screwed tightly and keep in fridge. Also take out in the car always, and keep cool in a thermos flask.

FRUITS:
Grapefruit, oranges, strawberries, (blackcurrants and blueberries and brambles for the good blue retinal pigments they contain.) 5 per day has been observed to be all some exceptional people need to reduce their arterial disease whilst young. Old age increases need for vitamin C.

GREENS:
Ideally raw e.g. broccoli, spinach, and the rest of the greens. Only avocados and bananas are fattening. For Olives it's best to buy whole olives and soak the salt   out.

LoSalt:
Worth having in the kitchen and car for when you have fish and chips out.
But chips not for the overweight. Potassium is more problem for people with weak hearts   .
Laxative
Sodium ascorbate powder. Used as a laxative; you find
the Laxative dose as determined by trial an error (3-13grms?) 6-7 am? 2 hrs before going out!
Take it in 1/2-3/4 oz or more of water for each gram. 1/2 to 1 gram (as tolerated) in every drink (not boiling) keep laxative dose + 1 or 2 grams by bedside to sip on retiring and if waking.
Vitamin C Rx is extremely variable according to results. Some people will live to 110 without ever taking vitamin C. Others will die young without extra.

The sodium in sodium ascorbate powder is very little absorbed. Most stays in the intestines when taking 3 or more grams. The sodium is less than 15% of the sodium ascorbate.

Vitamin E. (NATURAL)
1,000iu/day with main meal. If buying, avoid in capsules with soya or sunflower oil. Try to find it in glycerol. Raw sunflower oil is the best but rare.

Refined sunflower oil
is almost poisonous because the vitamin E has been destroyed so it can go rancid in the brain and arteries. That greatly increases the need for vitamin C and Vitamin E. D-alpha tocopherol is needed. The synthetic is 'dl'-alpha. NATURAL 'd'-alpha is essential. Synthetic 'dl' alpha could even be harmful.

L-Lysine powder
2 grams three times/day or a little less with every drink from age forty.(Incompatible with Alpha-Lipoic Acid - forms insoluble bond) so must be taken +/- 2 to 3 hrs before or after Lysine. Never investigated is why institutionalized, very old people survive without extra ascorbate and some excrete it on exclusion diets!

Co-Enzyme Q10
100 or 120mgs once/day (very variable according to results) at age 40. Ideally in capsules. Adding another capsule with every decade older seems sensible.

Alpha lipoic acid
Once/day and extra after any stomach upset or challenge to the liver (alcohol or any

toxin/infection) R form is best. Not with Lysine. Purpose is to protect liver and ability to detoxify toxins and recharges oxidised vitamin C.

100mgs at age 40 perhaps increasing with age. diabetic, are on thyroid medications, deficient in thiamine

Read more:
http://www.livestrong.com/article/517810-what-is-the-difference-in-r-alpha-lipoic-vs-alpha-lipoic-acid/#ixzz28q3SOYeW

Vitamin D3 2,000iu.

one or two day according to lack of sun exposure.
Selenium
200micrograms day
Ginkgo as directed on the bottle.
Fish oil (Omega 3) one capsule/day
Cod liver oil (1/day) (The small amounts of Ω 3 and vitamin D3 can be ignored.)
Glucosamine 1,000mg
Magnesium. Helps heart function.

All these should be taken as directed on labels.

If the skin of finger tips is hard - double the cod liver oil.

If joints - e.g. knees - ever cause a twinge, double the Glucosamine. If that doesn't stop it inside 48 hrs - double it again if you think you know what you were doing to damage your cartilages.

Please notify of any diagnosed illnesses and especially of colds and 'flu.' Dr Schallenberger MD., claims that his Ozone treatment cures arthritis.

The objective is not just to get you past 100 but without infirmity.

Overweight,

reduce it very gradually (1 lb per week maximum) before it reduces you.

Overweight and strong muscles can overload heart valves. Leaping up stairs two at a time may be easy for your legs but strains your mitral valve.

SLEEP

At least rest if you can't sleep. The Bible injunction to rest on the 7th day is essential advice for the healing of arteries and heart valves in Man with no inherent vitamin C manufacturing ability.

If you still can't do the Daily Mail 30 seconds challenge - add in your age?
Sydney Bush. HULL. Rev: 2nd May 2011.

WARNING
"Made with Butter!"

Don't believe it.
Look for the small print that includes vegetable oil!
Don't be surprised if you cannot find a supermarket bread, cake. pie or ready meal without it! Wonder why physicians don't do simple epidemiological studies to show the connection with cancer and type 2 Diabetes.

FRAUD

As the scandal grows in the USA surrounding Aspartame, people are now wondering how America was steamrollered into it. Could the cancer and other concerns, never materializing anywhere else in the world after 100 years safe use of saccharin, have been orchestrated to sell Aspartame – anything BUT safe?

Chapter V (Contributed by S.J. Bush)
Nutrition Relevant Eye Conditions

To begin with, a <u>short</u> list of curable and/ or greatly relieved illnesses simply using oral or intravenous vitamin C in most cases while arranging for referral.
Dr. Robert F. Cathcart MD always insisted that vitamin C was never wrong. Most of these conditions have been treated with vitamin C intravenously or orally by either Dr Klenner, Dr Cathcart or Dr Levy. (Dr. Fonorow's list)

Dr Klenner considered that every pathogenic virus could be killed by adequate vitamin C.
Here are more common Ocular disorders for which nutrition is expected to be relevant. It is not an exhaustive treatise on ocular pathology.
<u>Accommodation</u>: Weakness. See previous fortifying nutrition
Asthenopia can have origins in anaemia and malnutrition due to deficiencies of key vitamins.
<u>Age-related macular degeneration</u> — the photosensitive cells in the <u>macula</u> malfunction and over time cease to work. (There was marked improvement (attentuation of degenerative retinopathy) directly attributable to the vitamin C in this mouse model; All tested agents partially improved atrophic changes. Maeda T, Maeda A, et. al. *Evaluation of potential therapies for a mouse model of human age-related macular degeneration caused by delayed all-trans-retinal clearance.* Invest Ophthalmol Vis Sci. 2009 Jun 3 (See appendix peer reviewed papers)

Age Related Macular Degeneration Public Health Issue:

30% of Americans are affected (Taylor, Dorey and Nowell) and it is the primary cause of new blindness the vast majority being the 'Dry' type. Almost 90% of the blindness occurs in the 'wet' type – No clear link has been established but a link exists to lower socioeconomic groups suggesting that malnutrition is a factor.

Fruit and antioxidants are strongly indicated with – as a fire insurance, lutein and zeaxanthin plus many times daily ascorbate. This emerging disease is of rapidly increasing importance. My own most successful case – of the wet type, was restored to 90% vision in black and white after degenerating to the point where she could not see if the chart was switched on. Treatment was PDT at approx 10/20 followed by mega vitamins C, E and spinach.

Richer S and Stiles W, et al found with veterans, in 2011
1. "a larger percentage of Zeaxanthin (Zx) patients experienced clearing of their 10° Kinetic Visual Fields (KVF)central scotomas ($P = 0.057$). The "Faux Placebo" Lutein group was superior in terms of low-contrast visual acuity, CSF, and glare recovery, whereas Zx showed a trend toward significance." and
2. "Zeaxanthin induced foveal MPOD elevation mirrored that of Lutein and provided complementary distinct visual benefits by improving foveal cone-based visual parameters, whereas L enhanced those parameters associated with gross detailed rod-based vision, with considerable overlap between the 2 carotenoids. The equally dosed (atypical dietary ratio) Zx plus L group fared worse in terms of raising MPOD, presumably because of duodenal, hepatic-lipoprotein or retinal carotenoids competition. These results make biological sense based on retinal distribution

and Zx foveal predominance." Richer SP, Stiles W, et al., *Randomized, double-blind, placebo-controlled study of zeaxanthin and visual function in patients with atrophic age-related macular degeneration: the Zeaxanthin and Visual Function Study* (ZVF) FDA IND #78, 973. Optometry. 2011 Nov;82(11):667-680.e6. doi: 10.1016/j.optm.2011.08.008.

Amblyopia ('lazy eye,' often as 'lazy' as a broken leg. It is usually an overworked eye placing impossible demands on accommodation and convergence while retaining single binocular vision)) — poor or blurry vision due to no transmission or poor transmission of the visual image to the brain. Vitamin C is a neuro-transmitter. The original cause if due to alternating strabismus is unlikely to be significantly improved by nutrition. Vit C quickly cures and prevents measles, often the 'trigger' for strabismus.

Angioid streaks are a retinal condition characterized by breaks and cracks in Bruch's membrane. This is an outer retinal membrane transmitting nutrients to the retina. Bruch's membrane can thicken, become mineralised and lose its elasticity. All are likely to be improved or prevented by ascorbate.

Aniridia — a rare congenital eye condition leading to underdevelopment or even absence of the iris of the eye. Nothing can be expected to affect this condition during pregnancy. The condition has already been established by the genetic inheritance.

Anisometropia — the lenses of the two eyes have different focal lengths. It is an inherited condition impervious to nutritional treatments. The Bush Single power line free bicentric lens has been successfully employed to eliminate diplopia in translocating from distant to lower visual field, e.g. important when descending stairs and steps and looking down at instruments e.g. speedometer.

Antihistamines: While not being a disease except when in excess in the tissues, histamine is addressed by Western Medicine in completely the wrong way. Instead of the class of toxic drugs known collectively as 'Antihistamines' with every manufacturer seemingly in a race to get his own trial published, all that is needed is adequate vitamin C. It breaks down the histamine to harmless Hydantoin-5-acetic acid, water and carbon dioxide. This has, in the experience of Dr. Bush, the ability to virtually end complaints of 'dry eye' in a contact lens practice.

Anopsia. Vision loss – many causes. If due to any kind of encephalopathy, and especially if accompanied by fever, mega ascorbate is harmless and may resolve the condition.

Arc eye — a painful condition caused by exposure of unprotected eyes to bright light. Ascorbate drops and cod liver oil or a vitamin E capsule dripped into the eye are possible first aid measures.

Argyll Robertson pupil — small, unequal, irregularly shaped pupils Syphilitic in origin. Pupils react to accommodation but not to light. Intravenous vitamin C may cure the condition. Syphilis: Because there are some cases, intractable to antibiotics this may be an exception as regards being preventable? Curable? The author has seen no papers on this. Liposomal may cure or improve?
Atrophy of the Optic nerve in glaucoma is probably vascular and whilst damage may be irreversible, the

177

condition can probably be arrested with adequate ascorbate.

Blepharitis — inflammation of eyelids and eyelashes; characterized by white flaky skin near the eyelashes. Vitamins A, C and E are indicated.

Blepharochalasis. Due to life long stress of the orbicularis oculii muscles (usually in the absence of adequate spectacles) due to stretching and loss of elasticity of the palpebral skin.
f
Blindness — the brain does not receive optical information, through various causes. Underlying pathologies are many and, especially when caused by viral or bacterial infections. Virtually all viruses are killed by intravenous ascorbate.

Cataract — the lens becomes opaque, slowed if not prevented by antioxidants and UV protection. Vitamin C in the tears, cornea and aqueous, changes the wavelength of cataractogenic UVB to UVA. thereby also protecting the retina in addition to the absorptive retinal pigments. See End notes.

Central serous retinopathy is very likely to be preventable and due to occult scurvy. There appears to be a gender link. If so scurvy is a possible cause.

Chalazion cyst in usually the upper eyelid. Occult scurvy with vitamin E deficiency and oxidation of oils. Chorioretinal disorders. Mostly and very probably caused by prolonged, chronic occult scurvy

Chorioretinal Disseminated inflammation Mostly and very probably caused by chronic occult scurvy.

Chorioretinal inflammation in infectious and parasitic diseases. Vitamin C has cured Malaria Falciparum. Obviously IV ascorbate should be employed whatever other therapy is considered.

Choroidal haemorrhage: Mostly and very probably caused by prolonged, chronic occult scurvy.

Color blindness — Officially there is no known nutritional treatment. The single case of complete cure of macular degeneration by Dr. Bush from less than fingers to 20/15 after unsuccessful PDT, left the patient with black and white vision.

Conjunctivitis. Bacterial, viral. All types even U/V 'welders' flash' may be treated with dilute liposomal ascorbate directly into the eye and orally. But made with sodium ascorbate – NOT with ascorbic acid.

Conjunctivitis   Allergy   &   hyperemia   See Antihistamines

Corneal neovascularization. Mysterious condition associated with pterygium. Unknown cause.

Corneal ulcer. Guttae ascorbate especially for pseudomonas aeruginosa. Nakanishi (Japan) eliminated MRSA and PA with an ascorbate spray on burns. Antibiotics are potentiated and boils prevented.

Dacryoadenitis Mega-ascorbate to bowel tolerance and/or liposomal vitamin C. Antibiotics are potentiated.

Dermatitis of eyelid. Many causes Liposomal sodium ascorbate cannot ever be wrong.

(Leishmaniasis)
Sen G, Mukhopadhaya R, Ghosal J, Biswas T.
"Combination of ascorbate and alpha-tocopherol as a preventive therapy against structural and functional defects of erythrocytes in visceral leishmaniasis." Sen G, Mukhopadhaya R, Ghosal J, Biswas T. Free Radic Res. 2004 May;38(5):527-34
"Decreased hemoglobin (Hb) level was successfully replenished and was coupled with significant increase in the life span of red cells after treating the animals with both antioxidants. Results indicate better efficacy of the combination therapy with alpha-tocopherol and ascorbate in protecting the erythrocytes from structural and functional damages during leishmanial infection."

Diabetic retinopathy — damage to the retina caused by
complications of diabetes mellitus, which could eventually lead to blindness. Dice J.F., Daniel C.W.

The Hypoglycaemic effect of ascorbic acid in a juvenile onset diabetic. J. of the International Research Communications. 1: #4, 41, March 1973 (In this paper Dr Dice describes how he was diagnosed diabetic at age 15 and experimented on himself with vitamin C. between 7am and 1am he successfully reduced blood sugar by adding more "C" whenever glycosuria (sugar in the urine) occurred. When hypoglycaemia occurred, he lowered his insulin.

Three herbs figure in very hopeful and interesting research reported only in the last few days. These are rare and interesting developments in the novel research of Ren et al with vitamin D3. and Biswas, Chatterjee et al. using another herb of a tree

Strychnos potatorum Linn growing in Asia and Xu, Chen et al using Puerh Tea Polysacharides.

Last month yet another formal trial of Ayuverdic Indian medicine was also reported by Perez-Gutierrez et al. using the leaves of the Neem tree.

(Ren Z, Li W, Zhao Q, Ma L, Zhu J. The impact of 1,25-dihydroxy vitamin D3 on the expressions of vascular endothelial growth factor and transforming growth factor-β(1) in the retinas of rats with diabetes. Diabetes Res Clin Pract. 2012 Oct 19. pii: S0168-8227(12)00333-6. doi: 0.1016/j.diabres. 2012.09.028. Source: Department of Endocrinology, The First Affiliated Hospital of Xinjiang Medical University, Urumqi, China.
Biswas A, Chatterjee S, Chowdhury R, Sen S, Sarkar D, Chatterjee M, Das J. Antidiabetic effect of seeds of Strychnos potatorum Linn. in a streptozotocin-induced model of diabetes. Acta Pol Pharm. 2012 Sep-Oct;69(5):939-43.
Xu P, Chen H, Wang Y, Hochstetter D, Zhou T, Wang Y. Oral Administration of Puerh Tea Polysaccharides Lowers Blood Glucose Levels and Enhances Antioxidant Status in Alloxan-Induced Diabetic Mice. J. Food Sci.. 2012 Oct 11. doi: 10.1111/j.1750-3841.2012.
Perez-Gutierrez RM, Damian-Guzman M. Meliacinolin: A Potent α-Glucosidase and α-Amylase Inhibitor Isolated from Azadirachta indica Leaves and in Vivo Antidiabetic Property in Streptozotocin

Nicotinamide-Induced Type 2 Diabetes in Mice. Biol Pharm Bull. 2012;35(9):1516-24.

Drusen. Author has seen these disappear apparently with ascorbate.

Dystrophy, Corneal. No suggestions except best to evaluate g. ascorbate plus lyposomal whilst referring.

Ectropion Functional disorder unaffected by nutrition. See S.J. Bush. *"Non paralytic, Non spastic Ectropion."* Optometry Today. 1972

Entropion and trichiasis may be deficiency disease.

Epiphora Many causes.

Exophthalmos (Proptosis) Verma S, Sivanandan S, Aneesh MK, Gupta V, Seth R, Kabra S. Unilateral proptosis and extradural hematoma in a child with scurvy. Pediatr Radiol. 2007 Sep;37(9):937-9. Epub 2007 Jul 7 : Richardson O.B. Exophthalmos due to infantile scurvy. Bull. Acad. Med. Tor. 1948 Dec;22(3):51.

Exudative retinopathy
eyelid in herpes viral (herpes simplex) infection

Floaters — shadow-like shapes appearing singly or with others in the vitreous and field of vision

Glaucoma Bowel tolerance vitamin C (to achieve laxative effect via osmolarity if practical) and referral. Local conditions/ distance/ time etc., will decide.

Harada's disease Vogt-Koyanagi-Harada is a mysterious disease which needs referral but a harmless routine of liposomal vitamin C appears to be required if only from the point of view of zero risk to maximum possible benefit.

Histaminosis See Antihistamines.

Hordeolum ("stye" or "sty") — a bacterial infection of Sebaceous glands of eyelashes. (Occult scurvy).

Hollenhorst Microplaque Bifurcation blockage. Vit C

Hypertensive retinopathy — burst blood vessels, due to long-term high blood pressure of scorbutic origin,

Int ophthalmoplegia Eyelid involved other diseases

Iritis — inflammation of the iris: Mega ascorbate orally (see Acute Anterior Uveitis) guttae Sodium ascorbate with dilatation - and better still, liposomal ascorbic acid by mouth rather than 'ordinary sodium ascorbate or ascorbic acid. Hourly doses until referral to hospital achieved.

(Cyclitis is linked to iritis)

Irregular pupil. (No posterior synechiae) hypothesised as possibly due to being rooted in the vascular ciliary process in which vessel changes with occult scurvy will exert traction to distort the pupil simultaneously with changes in the trabeculum causing POAG.

Keratitis — inflammation of the cornea Mega ascorbate orally. G. Sodium ascorbate

Keratoconjunctivitis sicca — dry eyes Mega ascorbate orally. G. Sodium ascorbate and vitamin A.

Keratomycosis — fungal infection of the cornea lacrimal system. Various treatments have been used with ascorbate as adjunctive therapy.

Leprosy

Preventable? probably curable? No specific information Preventable? probably curable? No specific information due to medical obstruction. In humans the Mycobacterium Leprae targets skin around the eyes or anywhere and peripheral nerves. Not readily transmissible and virtually unresearched, another blot on the face of Western Medicine which might have found that 550 or 100 grams of ascorbate per day orally cures the disease. Dr. Thomas E. Levy has been extremely diligent in his search of the literature and found very many reports using miniscule amounts like 500mgs intramuscularly. Almost every report describes some improvement. 'Klenner size doses' would seem likely to offer a cure.

Macular degeneration — loss of central vision, due to macular degeneration: See Age Related Macular Degeneration.

Molluscum contagiosum Sufferers report high doses of vitamin C resolve it. If it is a virus then Klenner and many others would agree that ascorbate should kill it. However, the common small dermoid tumours so often seen do not always respond to mega vitamin C as sodium ascorbate. Perhaps they would if the vitamin were given in liposomal form. Since any attempt to produce a cure with liposomal C would not be injurious it is very worth the effort.

Nyctalopia (Nightblindness) — a condition making it difficult or impossible to see in the dark. Vitamin A may be deficient.

Onchocerciasis Obviously bowel tolerance C with any other therapy and ideally the liposomal form.
Ascorbate orally. G. Sodium ascorbate and vitamin A.

Ophthalmoparesis — the partial or total paralysis of the eye muscles Obviously mega C with any other therapy should be evaluated.

Optic disc drusen — globules progressively calcify in the optic disc, compressing the vasculature and optic nerve fibers, optic nerve and visual pathways Often seen to resolve with extra vitamin C.

Optic neuropathy - mega C with any other therapy. It is very noticeable that disc perfusion improves remarkably as soon as vitamin C is added into the diet

Pan-Uveitis - Preventable/curable by IV ascorbate or liposomal encapsulated ascorbate. Urgent referral. One expects this to be a primary disease of occult scurvy.

Peripheral retinal degeneration Mega nutrition. Nature protects the sight prioritising vitamin C to retina.

Posterior cyclitis Intravenous or liposomal vitamin C until referral achieved.

Presbyopia — a condition that occurs with growing age and results in the inability to focus on close objects. Vitamin C users often appear to delay it.

Primary open-angle glaucoma 'C' prevents/aborts?

Progressive external ophthalmoplegia — weakness of the external eye muscles. Mega nutrition.

Ptosis Adjunctive mega nutrition.

Red eye conjunctival hyperemia: typically due to

illness or injury. Bowel tolerance vit. C if mild.

Retinal detachment — the retina detaches from the choroid, leading to blurred and distorted vision
Bowel tolerance vitamin C for shock until urgent referral possibly for laser.

Retinal haemorrhage. Always bowel tolerance vitamin C with diabetic workup and referral.

Retinitis Always bowel tolerance vitamin C and E with diabetic workup.

Retinitis pigmentosa — genetic disorder; tunnel vision preceded by night-blindness. Blindness due to Bassen-Kornzweig syndrome can be prevented by vitamins E and A. (See Pauling: How To Live Longer and Feel Better 1986. p.280)

Retinoschisis Expected to improve with daily bowel tolerance vitamin C. the retina separates into several layers. Bowel tolerance vitamin C & Urgent referral.

River blindness — blindness caused by long-term infection by a parasitic worm (rare in western societies) Bowel tolerance and intravenous vitamin C as adjunctive therapies.

Scleritis — a painful inflammation of the sclera
Bowel tolerance vitamin C and referral.

Scorbutic Retinal detachments and breaks. If due to traction from increased tortuosity due to chronic occult scurvy, Adequate vitamin C and E expected to prevent recurrence when resolved. Retinal studies suggest that it is impossible to have increased tortuosity without detachment risk. Any mysterious fine lines appearing in the fundus photograph may predict retinal detachment. Disappear confirms.

Solar retinopathy. All antioxidants to prevent and repair damage due to solar burn.

Thygeson's superficial punctate keratopathy. Daily bowel tolerance ascorbate. G. Sodium ascorbate 5%. The fine spots at the limit of what can be observed in the blacked out consulting room can be obstinately difficult to resolve. Sometimes they persist for months.

Toxoplasma Bowel tolerance and IV ascorbate plus referral for urgent laser?

Tuberculosis. Liposomal vitamin C. Refer.

Uveitis — inflammatory process involving the interior of the eye; Bowel tolerance vitamin C immediately & urgent referral.

Urethritis – Because so much eye infection can be traced to Urethritis it is worth mentioning as a prevention, that as long as the urine is vitamin C rich, there is little chance of this.

Vitreous floaters. Avoid excess vitamin B2. Bowel tolerance vitamin C.

Xanthelasma of eyelid. Bowel tolerance vitamin C. The mysterious accumulations of lipd material in the eyelids are not understood and may be unrelated to total plasma cholesterol.

Xerophthalmia — dry eyes, caused by vitamin A deficiency. Can cause blindness.

<u>Yaws</u> Refer to dermatologist. Bowel tolerance C and liposomal vitamin C are suggested until referral.

Herpes <u>Zoster</u> Ophthalmicus L- Lysine, six grams, and bowel tolerance vitamin C (which appears to be a combination specific to the virus) until referral is achieved.

Dr. Cathcart always promoted the dictum – "You can never damage with extra vitamin C – only with too little!"

END NOTES:
Variations exist between the contractual obligations of Optometrists in different countries and states, re appropriate courses of action in the above, which are suggested as reasonable courses of action in most domains. Although orthomolecular physicians like the late Doctors Cathcart and Klenner, would have expected to treat many of the above conditions successfully with vitamin C (Cathcart Bowel Tolerance Table 1981) even before the advent of the liposomal form, the Optometrist is cautioned that nothing here is however, meant to override local or national custom and practice. Dr Thomas E. Levy MD.,JD., has described liposomal vitamin C as the 'Universal antidote.' Obviously there may be exceptions.

BassenKornzweig syndrome blindness due to this when caused by Retinitis Pigmentosa might be avoided with massive vitamins E and A.. (Pauling p 280 1st edn How to Live Longer and Feel Better)
Congenital cataract – exposure of mother to Rubella and Galactosaemia. Chron

Chapter VI
A Medical Hypothesis Rebuttal.

In this 'Review' we follow through an example of a typical, universal and apparently false medical hypothesis bringing misery to millions because knowledge of the benefits of multigram doses of vitamin C has been suppressed in medical school curricula. Dr. Bush contributes this chapter in the light of his own knowledge and experience from Nutritional CardioRetinometry®

=====

Terelak-Borys B, Skonieczna K, Grabska-Liberek I. Ocular ischemic syndrome - a systematic review. Med Sci Monit. 2012 Aug;18(8):RA138-144.

Abstract: Ocular ischemic syndrome is a rare condition, which is caused by ocular hypoperfusion due to stenosis or occlusion of the common or internal carotid arteries. Atherosclerosis is the major cause of changes in the carotid arteries. Ocular ischemic syndrome is manifested as visual loss, orbital pain and, frequently, changes of the visual field, and various anterior and posterior segment signs. Anterior segment signs include iris neovascularization and secondary neovascular glaucoma, iridocyclitis, asymmetric cataract, iris atrophy and sluggish reaction to light. Posterior eye segment changes are the most characteristic, such as narrowed retinal arteries, perifoveal telangiectasias, dilated retinal veins, mid-peripheral retinal hemorrhages, microaneurysms, neovascularization at the optic disk and in the retina, a cherry-red spot, cotton-wool spots, vitreous hemorrhage and normal-tension glaucoma.

189

Differential diagnosis of ocular ischemic syndrome includes diabetic retinopathy and moderate central retinal vein occlusion. Carotid artery imaging and fundus fluorescein angiography help to establish the diagnosis of ocular ischemic syndrome. The treatment can be local, for example, ocular (conservative, laser and surgical) or systemic (conservative and surgical treatment of the carotid artery). Since the condition does not affect the eyes alone, patients with ocular ischemic syndrome should be referred for consultation to the neurologist, vascular surgeon and cardiologist.

UNUSUALLY I would comment on this paper here before preparing a paper for that journal, the Medical Science Monitor, which I am not confident will be published. This is because it may be possible to show that "referral to neurologist, vascular surgeon and cardiologist" might be unnecessary in all these very common cases of the incipient, early condition, even in the most advanced – said here to be a 'rare' case.

 For every one of the above conditions and diagnoses, I believe there is a far simpler and better treatment. All the above conditions originate in occult scurvy. Let us take each condition and treatment in turn.
"Atherosclerosis is the major cause of changes in the carotid arteries."
"Ocular ischemic syndrome is manifested as visual loss, orbital pain and, frequently, changes of the visual field, and various anterior and posterior segment signs."

1.) "Anterior segment signs include iris neovascularisation" YES
2.) "and secondary neovascular glaucoma," Expected

3.) "iridocyclitis," YES
4.) "asymmetric cataract,"
5.) "iris atrophy and sluggish reaction to light." Expected
6.) "Posterior eye segment changes are the most characteristic, such as narrowed retinal arteries," YES
7.) "perifoveal telangiectasias," YES
8.) "dilated retinal veins," YES
9.) "mid-peripheral retinal hemorrhages, microaneurysms," YES
10.) "neovascularization at the optic disk and in the retina," YES
11.) "a cherry-red spot," NO
12.) "cotton-wool spots," YES
13.) "vitreous hemorrhage" YES
14.) "and normal-tension glaucoma." YES
15.) "Differential diagnosis of ocular ischemic syndrome includes diabetic retinopathy" YES
16.) "moderate central retinal vein occlusion."YES
17.) And lastly "surgical treatment of the carotid artery" to address a deficiency disease of scurvy.

Thus every single one of the above conditions can either be produced by chronic occult scurvy and reversed by vitamin C, or expected to be ameliorated however slowly, after prolonged vitamin C deficiency.

Photographic evidence for the reversal of the retinal vascular changes is plentiful, and diabetic changes in the retina were reversed as long ago as 1954 by Kempner. (KEMPNER W.

(*Radical dietary treatment of hypertensive and arteriosclerotic vascular disease, heart and kidney disease, and vascular retinopathy.* GP. 1954 Mar;9(3):71- 92.) Used by permission of Dr Bush)

For Notes

Note how although probably 80% of non-violent deaths are due to scurvy, directly or indirectly, the term becomes unacceptable and mentions of scurvy drop to near zero   soon after 1958. This concealed the danger of scurvy, already being suppressed. Did editors invite authors   to cooperate?

The refusals of the editors of the Journal of Medical Ethics and the British Medical Journal to let me publish the term 'Scurvy' suggest this?

The graph suggests that in 1958 there was no worry about publishing the term 'Scurvy.' But as more was learned about over fifty diseases being cured or prevented by vitamin C, a new threat to pharmacy and medical profits was perceived? Was strict information control then instituted to avert financial disaster due to the newly available vitamin C? If so the measures taken to protect the health of the PharMAFIA were a disaster for Mankind.

People had no defence against a "genocidal"* medical policy of sickness, carefully 'metered' in restrained milligrams of Vitamin C, whilst 'new' Hi-Tech image making drugs were produced for patents, profits and 'Medical Care.' e.g. the Statins. These in effect are a vitamin C substitute - to prevent. But they don't heal arteries like vitamin C. They kill!
* Drs. Hickey and Roberts.

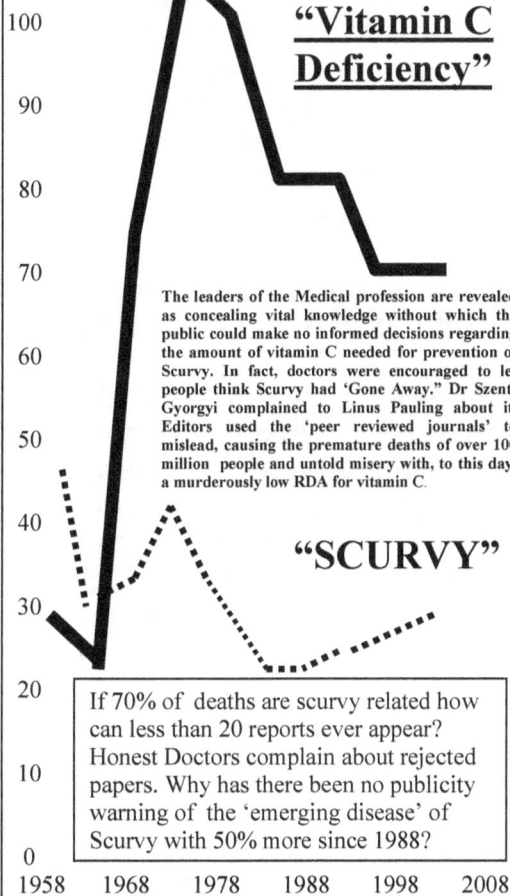

"Vitamin C Deficiency"

The leaders of the Medical profession are revealed as concealing vital knowledge without which the public could make no informed decisions regarding the amount of vitamin C needed for prevention of Scurvy. In fact, doctors were encouraged to let people think Scurvy had 'Gone Away." Dr Szent-Gyorgyi complained to Linus Pauling about it. Editors used the 'peer reviewed journals' to mislead, causing the premature deaths of over 100 million people and untold misery with, to this day, a murderously low RDA for vitamin C.

"SCURVY"

If 70% of deaths are scurvy related how can less than 20 reports ever appear? Honest Doctors complain about rejected papers. Why has there been no publicity warning of the 'emerging disease' of Scurvy with 50% more since 1988?

This graph was produced from the figures obtained from the National Library of Medicine search engine *PubMed* entering either "Scurvy" or "Vitamin C Deficiency" with AND followed by (Publication date. 1988) using 1988 in this example. An earlier search without (Publication Date) gave some accurate figures and then completely misleading results for later years. The graphed points represent the average annual papers in each five year period..

The massive increase in 'Vitamin C Deficiency' papers coupled with the significant increase in 'Scurvy' papers between 1967 and 1977 went unreported. Was the increase an arterfact of editorial policy and the 'news' perhaps 'managed' as the last 30 years papers suggest? If so, it is difficult to interpret except as a vile ill-health conspiracy now exposed.

Dissolved, the white streak down arteries and veins disappears, blood flow increases, vessels widen, the fundus darkens, pale areas disappear, acute bends and tortuosity of vessels disappears, risk of retinal detachment disappears, the disc becomes more pink, new, smaller vessels appear that had become sclerosed, cotton wool white spots of exudates disappear, drusen tend to disappear, the anterior adnexa lose their inflamed appearance as circumcorneal vessels shrink and the white sclera becomes the predominant feature.

Vessels in the conjunctiva become so faint and difficult to see that a microscope is needed.

It seems necessary to remind ourselves how far adrift medicine has become by re-reading the abstract to the above paper. What is wrong here is not the fault of the good doctors performing this research and coming to their honest conclusions. What is wrong is the curtailment of their education in medical school and the suppression of the information they need as shown by the graph. They had no chance against the system.

If we start with the statement "Atherosclerosis is the major cause of changes in the carotid arteries." This statement only appears to be a "which comes first the chicken or the egg" paradox. But there is no paradox. No illusion whatsoever. Pauling and Rath got it right.

Let us put it another way. Did the ambulance cause the accident? Surely it wouldn't have happened without its presence! That is the make believe cholesterol myth. Ambulances do not ordinarily cause accidents.

I will wager that even speeding as they often do, they are not responsible for a significant proportion of accidents in proportion to their number and miles traveled. But can there be any doubt that if the road were so badly maintained that the ambulance was thrown from side to side and could not negotiate a straight path, an accident becoming inevitable that would all change. The ambulance is innocent. The condition of the road is the problem. That is the basis of Pauling-Rath theory. There is no chicken and egg puzzle at all.

Arteries are not plastic tubes with smooth inner surfaces. Nature has constructed them from endothelial cells. Like the interwoven lacework of strengthening high tensile nylon or similar, around the garden hosepipe, arteries are strengthened by a meshwork of stringy collagen in three principal layers embedded in the wall of the artery. The artery is in poor condition because of lack of maintenance like the road. Its endothelial cells (road surface) are not being replaced due to lack of collagen. This may be due to lack of one or more of L-Lysine, Proline, Glycine, Vitamin C (Ascorbate.) instead of replacement cells to maintain the system watertight and prevent hydrolysis of the arterial adventitia in the basement membrane. Normally endothelial cells are firmly embedded in the basement membrane which is maintained as a healthy 'jelly-like' consistency. Scurvy changes the basement membrane from jelly to watery. It becomes more permeable to the aqueous component of the plasma and to lipid molecules which can infiltrate and pass more freely through it. Damaging collagen progressively in the tunicas intima, media and externa until the wall swells with blood pressure and pulse wave effects and is become aneurysmal.

Diastasis is the problem.

Separation of cells lining blood vessels, controlled by vitamin C maintaining the strength of the collagen which fastens cells together. (Gore et al. 1965) This may be the cause of the capillary fragility of scurvy. (Clemetson 1999) as the intercellular adhesion molecule-1 production decreases in scurvy. (Vincent HK, Bourguignon CM, Weltman AL, Vincent KR, Barrett E, Innes KE, Taylor AG. Effects of antioxidant supplementation on insulin sensitivity, endothelial adhesion molecules, and oxidative stress in normal-weight and overweight young adults. Metabolism 2009, Feb 58(2):254-62.)

"Ensheathment of vessels" is said to produce the arteriolar reflex

This is not so. Fats and cholesterol can and do penetrate into the tunica intima where they can become invaded by platelets, fibroblasts and macrophages. This causes swelling of the endothelial cell lined passageway through the length of the artery. But is not the 'ensheathment' taught in Optometry schools. It will certainly give rise to reflections, especially from the fats.

But as and when vitamin C and Lysine pass along the vessel their direct action both dissolves these substances which were helping the system remain watertight, helps to replace old and missing cells, and restores the lining of the vessel to prime condition in a circadian pattern of wear and tear made good.

Histamine
Additionally the Vitamin C is also acting to reduce the

higher plasma histamine levels extremely effectively – by as much as 70%. I am assured by practising physicians that this cannot be matched by any antihistamines at sub toxic levels. The manner in which vitamin C reduces plasma cholesterol is not taught in medical schools. It is interesting. Whereas all 'antihistamines' act on the hydrogen receptors

Monocyte adhesion
Clemetson in his monocyte adhesion theory of heart disease suggests monocytes – white cells in the plasma 'sticking' more readily to the endothelial lining of the vessels when histamine levels are high as plasma ascorbate falls. Clemetson published his paper in Medical Hypotheses because of the anti-vitamin C bias of the leading journals, the Journal of the American Medical Association being the most prominent. Linus Pauling rightly complained in his last book about the selective nature of the Journal of the American Medical Association, an unreliable journal for anything to do with scurvy or vitamin C, publishing, as he pointed out, only negative articles. It is likely that to this day, US doctors believe they might cause anaemia by prescribing vitamin C because spurious work by well known anti-vitamin researcher Vincent Marks' article was published but no correction was permitted. The correction had to be published in journals that JAMA's readers were unlikely to read. This is one more example of the conspiracy against vitamin C and scurvy. Clemetson claimed that Diastasis, a separation of the endothelial cells lining the arteries, allows penetration by the plasma (under blood pressure) leading to cholesterol and monocyte adhesion. It does not differ greatly in principle from Pauling/Rath theory, both placing deficiency of vitamin C as a prerequisite for the initiation of atherogenesis. It was developed further

by other researchers after Clemetson's paper. Clemetson CA. The key role of histamine in the development of atherosclerosis and coronary heart disease. Med Hypotheses. 1999 Jan;52(1):1-8. Histamine and ascorbic acid in human blood. J Nutr. 1980 Apr;110(4):662-8. Clemetson forged the link between sleep lack (stress) and the rise of histamine with the concomitant pathology associated with scurvy.

Clemetson is noteworthy for the vast amount of pure research he performed on vitamin C also writing about abruptio placentae. His large volumes are difficult to obtain but are classics and probably increasing in value.

Majno and Palade's earlier work is noteworthy, for in 1961 they demonstrated separation of the endothelial cells using the electron microscope. Majno G, Palade GE, Schoefl GI Studies on inflammation II. The site of action of histamine and serotonin along the vascular tree: a topographical study. Biophys Biochem Cytol. 1961 Dec;11:607-26. Levy T.E. believes that this is a key element in the development of porosity of the system and for cholesterol to be laid down.

Some notes on Pauling Rath Theory and Haemodynamics
The pulse wave and surge in pressure every second stretch the endothelial cells. The aqueous phase of the plasma is never under less than the diastolic pressure, and double that, with exertion. Some idea of the force applied by the heart to the blood flow can be obtained from an attempt to blow the mercury out of a 'U' tube. If you can produce a difference of levels of over 12mms you will be doing well!

Cells that were not ready to be replaced can be torn away and leave an exit for water under much pressure. This would 'ungel' the collagen, make the arterial wall soggy and destroy its strength.

The very low density cholesterol Lp(a) is found in Man and Guinea Pig and the very few other supramarine animals, Indian Fruit eating bat, Red Vented Bul-Bul and some primates that don't make significant amounts of vitamin C unlike all the other creatures having little very low density lipoprotein alpha type of cholesterol.

This is attracted to the injured site of the arterial wall as the cholesterol washes over lysil strands from damaged tissues locking into the lysil binding sites on the Apo(a) molecule of the lipoprotein alpha component of plasma unique to anascorbaemic species.

Thus [Lp(a)] is brought close to the damaged sites and impacts making a waterproof seal. Additionally, low vitamin C and E have been shown to accompany inflammatory arterial response with raised C-reactive protein and intercellular adhesive molecule supporting Clemetson's histamine involvement. (Tahir M, Foley B, Pate G, Crean P, Moore D, McCarroll N, Walsh M. Impact of vitamin E and C supplementation on serum adhesion molecules in chronic degenerative aortic stenosis: a randomized controlled trial. Am Heart J. 2005 Aug;150(2):302-6.)

There is little doubt that Pauling/Rath and Clemetson's theories of atherosclerosis are mutually supportive, both heavily dependent on antioxidants in general and vitamin C in particular. Dr. Matthias Rath who survives Linus Pauling, helped formulate this theory and calls this a metabolic countermeasure. A thicker arterial wall is what he describes as a genetic countermeasure to the lack of vitamin C which is at a constantly higher level in all other animals which is why they do not develop arterial disease unless e.g., feeding rabbits with butter. Mice deprived of their vitamin C gene, quickly die of heart attack if not fed large amounts of vitamin C.

This is because mice do not possess an erythrocyte glucose1 transporter (GLUT1) as they never needed one, being able to generate ascorbate as necessary.

Our remarkable blood! Montel-Hagen, Sitbon and Taylor, clever researchers, commented on the "assumption always having been made that the blood of all mammalian species behaved in the same way." Now we know that in breeding the vitamin C knockout mouse, a species was created that cannot be expected, in the wild, to acquire adequate dietary vitamin C. Many doctors in the "anti-vitamin C" camp refuse to recognise this which is how, by restricting the knowledge, 'official,' or 'Western medicine,' maintains a prolific array of preventable disease (as displayed above) for lifelong 'management' by an ever increasing array of 'specialists.'

Without imposed ignorance and a genocidal RDA for vitamin C medical fortunes would rapidly wane and there would be no vast world-wide coronary artery bypass business. The Pauling Rath theory was published in 1990, with variations since then and won patents on the dissolving of plaque (mixture for cholesterol oxidised cholesterol calcium and plasma components) using nothing more than improved ratios of the nutrients found naturally in the blood stream. That is what defines Orthomolecular Medicine; making the plaque go back where it came from.

==================================

Dr. Vincent Marks:
No serious work on nutrition would be complete without reference to this man. We owe him a great deal for his patient and persistent earning of notoriety for his valuable emphasis on the dangers of vitamins, where few would fear to tread. Unable to find any deaths, he still performs sterling service in this respect. He is a learned and valorous professor of biochemistry and frequently alerts us to the dangers of vitamin C. I quote Martin J. Walker MA. author of the compulsive reading 730 pages "Dirty Medicine." I do not want to be sued by Dr. Marks who is well known for this which is why I quote Martin Walker an authority on conflicts of interest in the medical profession's leading members serving on influential committees liaising with the food industry and pharmacy.
Taken from http://www.whale.to/a/marks1.html

The choice of title for the booklet is interesting; the use of 'British' in the title immediately deflects the argument of most contemporary critics of processed food. Another less misleading title like 'Is Industrially Produced Food Bad For You?' would have engendered quite a different debate. In fact the booklet does not actually apply itself to the issue of British food, except in a couple of cases where, by implication, Marks argues against himself: on BSE for instance, 'So far the occurrence of BSE in other countries has not been reported'.
The first twelve pages comprise an assault upon those who do not share Marks' views on industrially produced foodstuffs. In these pages he manages to

201

touch upon all the favourite targets of the Campaign Against Health Fraud. Of those who feel uncomfortable with the involvement of industrially-funded science in food production, Marks says:

These, mainly middle-class, scientifically ill-informed individuals feel more comfortable with things that are naively or exploitatively referred to as 'natural' - without understanding quite what that term means - than they are with products they perceive as being manufactured or synthetic.

Such scathing and irrational attitudes have no place in a serious text, especially from someone who purports to be a scientist. Marks however seems to enjoy this kind of populist harangue. As he moves from the scientifically specific to the pathologically general, his science turns to ideology.

Perhaps at this point we should look at what the Institute of Medicine's Dietary Reference Intake manual states. More reasonably on page 402 they say in a section on major knowledge gaps, discussing depletion and repletion periods for vitamin C "The depletion and repletion periods should be sufficiently long to allow a new steady state to be reached. This can be very problematic for vitamin C because the biological half-life ranges from 8 to 40 days and is inversely related to the ascorbate body pool.

Bush: It gets worse
"For Beta carotene and other carotenoids, no long term depletion-repletion studies with validated intermediate end points exist."

Our most expert physicians inform us then in this major reference work, that "For vitamin C, vitamin E,

Selenium and Beta Carotene and other carotenoids, useful data are seriously lacking for setting requirements for infants, adolescents, pregnant and lactating women, and the elderly."

We knew after 2004, from Hickey and Roberts that the quite ridiculous RDA for vitamin C was a joke with over 100 childish errors in its determination and about fifty more that I suggest in the encyclopaedia.

Gender issues are addressed in the statement – "Data are lacking about gender issues with respect to metabolism and requirements for these nutrients. For example, women and children with low intakes of selenium are at higher risk of Keshan disease than are men with similar intakes. Women are at higher risk of macular degeneration even at similar plasma concentrations of carotenoids.

Now for the really scary admissions.

"The understanding of the health effects of carotenoids is rudimentary compared with the other nutrients in this report. Little information is available on bioavailability, toxicity and effects of these compounds apart from Beta carotene. (NOTE! and they made a terrible mistake abandoning the Finnish study which people still quote wrongly as linking Beta carotene with lung cancer.)

These experts then continue "Although the only known validated function of carotenoids in humans is to act as a source of vitamin A in the diet, little is known about the relative contribution of dietary provitamin A carotenoids to vitamin A status.

I am sorry to say that the threat to life from this lack of information gets worse as we read the text on page 404 regarding vitamin E and I recommend Andreas Papas' book for more information on vitamin E.

With what I can only view as callous disregard for public health, these authors ignore the dangers from modern culinary polyunsaturated oils which are deadly to one's vitamin E and total antioxidant status.

These Institute authors state – quite unbelievably – "Research to date has indicated very little cause for concern about the adequacy of vitamin E intake for apparently healthy people;" (who knows? A girl was found who lived on doughnuts deep fried in 'vegetable' oil.)

They continue stating "A growing number of studies suggest that there are complex interrelationships between nutrients, particularly those involved in protecting against oxidation e.g. vitamins C and E and Selenium."

Then they have the effrontery to continue with the statement – as if it cannot really be very important,

but these are not well understood in relation to the maintenance of normal nutritional status and to the prevention of chronic degenerative disease. These interactions may affect the intake level for one or more of the nutrients." So although they are not understood they gamble with people's lives.

Linus Pauling was the most revered of American scientists. He stopped atmospheric testing of atom bombs and prevented countless cancers. He stressed the mutually supportive roles of vitamins C and E and emphasised how "a diet high in unsaturated fatty acids, especially the polyunsaturated ones, can destroy the body's supply of vitamin E and cause muscular lesions, brain and degeneration of blood vessels. Care must be taken not to include a large amount of polyunsaturated oil in the diet without a corresponding increase in vitamin E. Unsurprisingly; Adele Davis said the same thing back in 1966.

Can it possibly get worse? Yes. Large scale epidemiological number crunching of physicians and nurses histories takes little account of what kind of vitamin E was used. The natural is many times more effective than artificial type, and when more specialised double blind studies are carried out, the wrong vitamin E has been found to justify negative coordinated newspaper headlines about the vitamin E. In short, whatever negative report is published about either vitamin C or E is best binned. It is increasingly obvious that just as Prof. Richard Smith stated that "The peer reviewed medical journals have become a marketing extension of the pharmaceutical industry," that industry has moved on to make the newspapers serve in the same role. One large circulation UK newspaper, well known for its weekly well known 'Health Section" mentions vitamin C about four times per year. Recently a double page spread devoted to cancer failed to mention vitamin C once and heart/stroke articles rarely.

How much of a threat is vitamin E seen to represent to medicine and pharmacy? Note the recent reduction of the RDA despite all protests. Without any proper evidence, it was simply reduced to an amount posing less threat to pharmaco-medical profits.

Undoubtedly, from their own mouths, our medical leaders are reckless and uncaring in their attitude of limiting recommended amounts of nutrients, long established as harmless. Indeed they give the game away with the published tables for Das, Dey and Ghosh et al. In Calcutta, India in 2012 found very convincingly, that supplementary vitamin "C may be a novel and simple therapy for the prevention of pathological cardiovascular events in habitual smokers."

In the USA Pauling and Rath were again supported by Liu and Meydani who showed in 2002 that progressive arteriosclerosis after heart transplant could be retarded by vitamin C and E using the intravascular ultrasound technique,

Do antioxidants extend life?

I had to laugh. The Institute of Medicine's statements were so gloomy but there was honey in the tail. At the end of the book tables show the amounts of vitamins C, E, A and Selenium in the plasma of people in every age group up to the 90s.

Would you believe it? The highest plasma concentrations of all the nutrients, vitamins C, E Selenium, Lycopene and carotenoids were in the oldest! Does that tell us something?

Chapter VII
Vitamin C – Eye Opening History!

Vitamin C is not really a vitamin. It is a co-enzyme. Irwin Stone called it the missing stress hormone.

Vitamin C and cholesterol are inextricably interrelated. The statin medication works through the same pathway as vitamin C in the liver, in controlling plasma cholesterol. But whereas the statins cause a multitude of disabling and potentially fatal adverse effects, vitamin C causes none whatever.

When coronary thrombosis started killing people, physicians appeared useless and were widely scorned when they too succumbed to heart attacks. A great loss of confidence beset medicine. There were no antibiotics. Sulfonamides were useless. The Spanish Flu had killed millions. Herbalists were often more highly regarded. Frightened of losing what bit of credibility they had to vitamin C and fearing that unless they found a cause for the coronary thrombosis they latched on to the saturated fat and cholesterol myth boosted by David Kritchevsky. He was to change his opinions later, but his distorted paper and graphs omitting the statistics that did not fit, were influential in swaying physicians.

Drugs were produced with the claim that they would lower cholesterol and end the epidemic. They didn't.
Linus Pauling was embroiled unexpectedly in argument about it, and being the foremost chemist in

the world, he felt challenged to explore the subject. Even more unexpectedly, he found massive opposition from the physicians of "Official Medicine."

His own son a physician, and others, were honest. But dishonesty reigned in the US as in the UK and all Western Medical Schools. Eventually Cathcart, Denham Harman, Abram Hoffer and a nucleus of honest physicians tried to overcome the block but couldn't.

So powerful is the medical opposition to vitamin C (as with vitamin E - could they know more than we do – it appears so – why else should they reduce the RDA for non-toxic vitamin E?) that Pauling only managed to penetrate the anti-vitamin C shield with two peer reviewed papers having had hundreds published on chemical themes. As the only man to win two unshared Nobel prizes he could not break down the wall of PharmacoMedical defence.

Eventually, just as a disgusted Dr. Klenner scolded his colleagues, saying they preferred to allow people to die rather than admit the power of vitamin C, Pauling is quoted in similar fashion. On the back cover of Rath's "Why Animals Don't Get Heart Attacks but People Do!" Pauling says to Rath, after years of them working together and writing the Unified Theory of Heart Disease,

> "Your discoveries are so important for millions of people that they threaten entire industries. One day there may even be wars just to prevent this breakthrough from being widely accepted. This is the time when you need to stand up."

Aided by cardiologist Matthias Rath and Scottish physician Dr. Ewan Cameron, curing about 15% of cancers in Scotland and whose results almost perfectly paralleled the success of Morishige and Murata in Japan he grew more interested in Medicine. He taught the physicians the fundamentals of sickle cell disease but still, they tried to ignore him.

He became fixated against the opposition. Eventually he broke away from Arthur Robinson over perhaps unfortunate misunderstandings and the finding that in the case of hairless mice and squamous cell carcinoma, vitamin C did not always suppress cancer but, very oddly, in the experiment, actually seemed – at intermediate dosages, to stimulate it. Now we know from Montel-Hagen, Sitbon and Taylor that animal models might be completely misleading. This is how they put it when they published their review in May 2009 – causing red faces in many laboratories –

On the basis of human data, it was assumed that all mammalian erythrocytes express GLUT1 and that this transporter functions similarly in red cells of different species.

RECENT FINDINGS:
Analyses of erythrocytes from diverse mammalian species showed that GLUT1 is restricted to those few mammals who are unable to synthesize ascorbic acid from glucose comprising higher primates, guinea pigs, and fruit bats.

Sadly, Pauling's wife and former student Ava Helen died of gastric cancer and Pauling was destined to die of prostatic cancer. Since then Dr Rath carrying on with Pauling's research, found that bioflavonoids as in Chinese Green Tea, could produce an anticancer effect and pharmacologists Prof. Steve Hickey and Dr. Hilary Roberts feel that vitamin K is also involved in a cure. Readers have to study the work of Rath, Hickey and Roberts in their books remembering the difficulty of finding suppressed vitamin C research in the archive of Official Medicine. This vastly devalues PubMed as a serious resource of useful knowledge.

Knowing this one starts to look deeper. We examine the titles of the thousands of papers published in recent years in relation to vitamin C, ascorbic acid, sodium ascorbate, antioxidants, vitamin E, and particularly examine those that are meant to impress the public such as Physicians and Nurses studies on thousands of them. Are they reliable? Do they use the optimal quantities? Do they even guarantee to use effective forms of the nutrients? Could they actually be using relatively useless synthetic vitamin E?

Whilst physicians most commonly prescribe water soluble drugs to be taken four times per day for maximum effect is vitamin C ever prescribed that way?

Unfortunately rigorous examination of methods and results show that too often, benefits are minimal and the data we want is missing.

Worse than this is Pauling's finding. He listed 16 medically controlled trials of vitamin C in common studies in his 1986 book. They showed very impressive benefits. Four of the sixteen studies resulted in 50% or more reduction of illness. The average of all the studies few using as much as 1 gram of vitamin C, was 34%. Read any report today and these figures are denigrated.

Read reports of the Cochrane Library and other influential bodies and one is left feeling that there is an incorrespondence of views and others as beyond the scope of this book.

The Institute of Medicine's manual of Dietary Reference Intakes again, is a very important reference.

With unaccustomed frankness, the DRI manual of 2000, states "- - -there are wide uncertainties in the data used to estimate vitamin C requirements. However in the absence of other data, maximal neutrophil concentration with minimal urinary loss appears to be the best biomarker at the present time. It must be emphasised that research is urgently needed to explore the use of other biomarkers to assess vitamin C needs."

In view of this position statement, Hickey and Roberts, having become aware of CardioRetinometry®, contacted Bush in order to verify the adrenaline like action of ascorbate on blood vessels in the anterior eye – the circumcorneal plexus. Bush was able, even before Prof Hickey suggested it, to offer that he had associated an adrenaline like effect with his observations which were based on slit lamp biomicroscopy of corneal and other reactions to contact lens wearing. But Pharmacy beholden Optometry journals would not publish this information.

Bush advised Hickey that the arteriolar reflex was not as thought, and that what he was seeing could only be explained as supporting Pauling Rath theory of the dissolving of ageing arterial blockages (Atheroma)

Hickey and Roberts then went to press with images of circum-corneal blood vessels disappearing after extra vitamin C, claimed by patients as taken following the advice and the making available of 200 gram pots of sodium ascorbate. Pauling used ascorbic acid. Bush preferred sodium ascorbate as the more alkaline - especially if there could be doubt about acidity encouraging cancer.

Hickey and Roberts book was then published in 2004, devoting almost the entire chapter on "Quantifiable biomarkers for scurvy" (Pp107-11) to what was later described on the Cosmopolitan University website newsletter, as Bush's new science. Hickey and Roberts described it as providing "a new technique for estimation of vitamin C requirements.", thus stating that "this effect may provide a more rigorous derivation of intake requirements." And went on to quote Bush as formulating a

> 'preliminary redefinition of scurvy as –"any state in which supplemental vitamin C improves the pericorneal vasculature"'

and quoted Bush as saying that "the retinal blood vessels improved in over 90% of patients taking high dose vitamin C." Hickey and Roberts then confirmed that the observation is consistent with the claims of Pauling and others for heart disease as scurvy.

For more detail on the chemistry of vitamin C, a subject growing by the day, the reader must consult the appropriate texts. This entire book could not cover a quarter of it. Years ago Clemetson published a massive tome and more recently Lester Packer and Jürgen Fuchs performed a great service bringing us the

work of Howerde Sauerblich (History of vitamin C)
Constance S. Tsao (Biochemistry)

Barry Halliwell, Mathew Whiteman (Antioxidant and
prooxidant properties of vitamin C)
Wolf Bors, Garry Buettner (The Vitamin C Radical
and its Reactions)

Lester Packer himself (Vitamin C and Redox Cycling
Antioxidants)

William W. Wells, Che-Hun Jung (Regeneration of
vitamin C)

Beryl J Ortwerth, Vincent M. Monnier (Protein
Glycation by the Oxidation Products of Ascorbic
Acid)

Richard C. Rose, John X. Wilson (Ascorbate
Membrane Transport Properties)

Balz Frei (Vitamin C as an Antiatherogen:
Mechanisms of action)

Etsuo Niki, Noriko Noguchi ((Protection of Human
Low Density Lipoprotein from Oxidative
Modification by Vitamin C)

Alan Anthony Woodall, Bruce N. Ames (Diet and
Oxidative Damage to DNA: The Importance of
Ascorbate as an Antioxidant)

Charles L. Phillips, Heather N. Yeowell (Vitamin C,
Collagen Biosynthesis, and Aging)

Allen Taylor, C. K. Dorey, Thomas Nowell (Oxidative
Stress and Ascorbate in Relation to Risk for
Cataract and Age-Related Maculopathy)

Lou Ann S. Brown, Dean P. Jones (Antioxidant Action of Vitamin C in the Lung)

Gary E. Hatch (Vitamin C and Asthma)

Hans-Anton Lehr, Rainer K. Saetzler, Karl E. Arfors (Effect of Vitamin C on Leucocyte Function and Adhesion to Endothelial Cells)

Raxit J. Jariwalla, Steve Harakeh (Mechanisms Underlying the Action of Vitamin C in Viral and Immunodeficiency Disease)

Daniel Tsun-Yee Chiu, Mei-Ling Cheng (Blood Vitamin C in Human Glucose-6-Phosphate Dehydrogenase Deficiency)

Jürgen Fuchs, Maurizzio Podda (Vitamin C in Cutaneous Biology)

Betty Jane Burri, Robert A. Jacob (Human Metabolism and the Requirement for Vitamin C)

Adriann Bendich (Vitamin C Safety in Humans)

James E. Enstrom (Vitamin C in prospective Epidemiological Studies)

Jason P. Eiserich, Carroll E Cross, Albert Van der Vliet (Nitrogen Oxides are Important Contributors to Cigarette Smoke-Induced Ascorbate Oxidation)

Ching K. Chow (Vitamin C and Cigarette Smoke)

Ritva Järvinen, Paul Knekt (Vitamin C, Smoking, and Alcohol Consumption)

215

Chapter VIII
Conclusion

By way of review let's look at the pathway and to road signs in our quest to be the most effective health care professionals. The basics of good health are good nutrition and life style. Many abuse their bodies for long years and expect their doctor to correct, by a pill, injection or surgery, what they have created over a long period of time.

As health care professionals we are obligated to help our patients not only in their present distress but to educate them for better health down the path of life. That means teaching them how to manage their own health while you are applying all that you know in your profession as an eye care specialist, to rectify the problem and restore good vision. Since procedures for vision appointments take up so much of the Optometrists time it would be helpful to have a brochure on hand to give to patients so that they can control their own destiny for ocular health.

When troubles come, as they do, even when we try our best for good health in a polluted world, we need to know the four basics of Nourishment, Oxygen, Exercise and Balancing it all, for spectacular results.

Then with this comes the opportunity to offer your patients, the best possible protection against the most common cause of death by heart attacks or strokes through CardioRetinometry®.

This marvelous discovery by Dr Sydney Bush, has been tried, tested and documented in "before and after photos", of the vascular structure in the interior of the eye, in hundreds of patients and is without question the only form of treatment that guarantees success against these killer diseases.

The most common eye diseases in the western world are cataract, glaucoma, macular degeneration or holes, retinal tears and detachment, etc. If the eye care professionals can alleviate suffering in these alone there would be less blindness in the western world. If we can clear the arterioles and veins in the eyes, we can prevent much eye disease and blindness just by the fact of getting the nutrients to the eyes.

As Dr. Hedahl said at my last visit, "Whatever is good for the heart is good for the eyes." So it is like a double bonus to follow good nutrition for both. This is substantiated by Dr. Bush with CardioRetinometry®.

Eye diseases in the third world countries are rampant and blindness is common. Besides being nutritionally deficient, people are largely infected with due to poor sanitation and primitive living conditions, many drinking from waters that are known to give them parasites. I have seen photos of people picking worms out of their thigh skin, after drinking the only water available to them. Ministries that are providing good water wells for communities are doing a great service to mankind.

As we look toward improving vision, we must make our protocols easy for patients to follow. That is the one thing that all health care professionals deal with, i.e., patient compliance. Often what seems so easy to us, because we know the reasons behind the treatment, yet the patient has a difficult time being consistent. It is our task to make that easier for them. It can be done with simple daily dose charts that can be filled out for each patient so they can refer to it often as they find their way to health and restoration.

 Another help is to have on hand some basic booklets or brochures explaining the procedures to which they can refer. Also books of good health practices can be recommended or kept in the waiting area to encourage further education. It is less surprising nowadays how many people would rather read something like that, than to read about a movie star's latest escapade into immorality or a major sport achievement.

I am not downplaying social interests, but we healthcare professionals can educate people too, just as the media does with their interests. We simply need to recognise that patients are likely now to display increasing trust in Optometrists to keep them well, rather than physicians to get them better!

The supplements we recommend must be easy to obtain, preferably at one site. Dr Bush has for many years registered Hearteries® for his nutrients, but has not developed it as he does not want to be a vitamin salesman. He may eventually make them available directly from his Institute.

Chiropractors are now ordering natural supplements for their patients as Nutritionists have done for years.

It is my hope that Optometrists will follow suit. Incorporating these good antioxidants and eye supplements has a risk to benefit ratio that makes it virtually criminal not to counsel and dispense for at least macular degeneration prevention. Taking these nutrients into their practices ensures the quality and value our patients deserve.

APPENDIX (1)

Trachoma: the leading cause of blindness

This is taken from the World Concerns website which covers many health conditions among them blindness from lack of good nutrition, sanitation and water supply.

Trachoma: the leading cause of preventable blindness, affects over 35 million people, yet is often easily preventable if not for poverty. (Robert Semeniuk, Personalizing the World Health Crisis.)

This is just a small example. There are many more1 diseases and deteriorating health systems which cost many, many lives each year.

Poverty and social conditions, brought upon by human decisions and global institutions to shape the world economy in a way that favours a few western countries to the detriment of the rest of the world, continue. Increased poverty and debt is resulting in forced cut-backs in health and education, the very things that would help form a foundation in ensuring such impacts are minimized.

Many news reports and much coverage tends to be of stock markets, booming (or now receding) economics, international war on terrorism, a few other selected conflicts and local news. One issue that is often missed or suppressed by the mainstream media is the sheer number of people affected and dying from tropical and infectious diseases— largely preventable and curable especially by vitamin C alone.

The poorest countries in the world will always suffer compared with the richest. Eleven million people in poor countries will die from infectious diseases this year. By the time you finish reading this column 100 people will have died. Half of them will be children aged under five.
— Larry Elliott, Evil triumphs in a sick society Guardian, February 12, 2001

BISPHENOLS
Another concern is plastic packaging and the endocrine disruptor bisphenol, leaching from it. Baby feeding bottles must not contain it and they are regulated. The linings of cans however are suspect. Ocular complications can reasonably be expected eventually.

The scandal of marketing formula milk is well known.

APPENDIX (2)

Resumés from some of the most important peer reviewed citations - mostly PubMed.

Richer SP, Stiles W, Graham-Hoffman K, Levin M, Ruskin D, Wrobel J, Park DW, Thomas C. *Randomized, double-blind, placebo-controlled study of zeaxanthin and visual function in patients with atrophic age-related macular degeneration: the Zeaxanthin and Visual Function Study (ZVF) FDA IND #78, 973.*

Optometry. 2011 Nov;82(11):667-680.e6. doi: 10.1016/j.optm.2011.08.008.

"The purpose of this study is to evaluate whether dietary supplementation with the carotenoid zeaxanthin (Zx) raises macula pigment optical density (MPOD) and has unique visual benefits for patients with early atrophic macular degeneration having visual symptoms - - - In older male patients with AMD, Zx-induced foveal MPOD elevation mirrored that of L and provided complementary distinct visual benefits by improving foveal cone-based visual parameters, whereas L enhanced those parameters associated with gross detailed rod-based vision, with considerable overlap between the 2 carotenoids. The equally dosed (atypical dietary ratio) Zx plus L group fared worse in terms of raising MPOD, presumably because of duodenal, hepatic-lipoprotein or retinal carotenoid competition. These results make biological sense based on retinal distribution and Zx foveal predominance."

=================================

Rizzo MR, Abbatecola AM, Barbieri M, Vietri MT, Cioffi M, Grella R, Molinari A, Forsey R, Powell J, Paolisso G

Evidence for anti-inflammatory effects of combined administration of vitamin E and C in older persons with impaired fasting glucose: impact on insulin action. J Am Coll Nutr. 2008 Aug;27(4):505-11. Comment: Vitamins E and C lowered inflammation and improved insulin action through a rise in non-oxidative glucose metabolism.

================================

Nutr Rev. 2002 Nov;60(11):368-71.
Combined vitamin C and E supplementation retards early progression of arteriosclerosis in heart transplant patients. Liu L, Meydani M.
Source
Vascular Biology Laboratory, Jean Mayer USDA Human Nutrition Research Center on Aging at Tufts University,
Comment: Vitamins C and E retarded the progression of coronary arteriosclerosis.

================================

Gökkusu C, Palanduz S, Ademoğlu E, Tamer S.
Oxidant and antioxidant systems in niddm patients: influence of vitamin E supplementation. Endocr Res. 2001 Aug;27(3):377-86.
Comment: Long-term studies are needed to demonstrate the beneficial effects of vitamin E on treatment/prevention of NIDDM."

================================

Das A, Dey N, Ghosh A, Das S, Chattopadhyay DJ, Chatterjee IB. Molecular and cellular mechanisms of cigarette smoke-induced myocardial injury: prevention by vitamin C. PLoS One. 2012;7(9):e44151. Epub 2012 Sep 6. 2012

Source
Department of Biotechnology, Dr. B. C. Guha Centre for Genetic Engineering and Biotechnology, Calcutta University College of Science, Kolkata, India.
Comment: Vitamin C may be a novel and simple therapy for the prevention of pathological cardiovascular events in habitual smokers.

===
Am J Cardiol. 2003 Aug 1;92(3):334-6.
Relation of aggressiveness of lipid-lowering treatment to changes in calcified plaque burden by electron beam tomography.

Hecht HS, Harman SM.
Source
Beth Israel Medical Center, New York, New York 10003, USA. hhecht@aol.com
Comment: Regarding LDL cholesterol lowering, "lower is better" is not supported by changes in calcified plaque progression.
================================
Garcia-Bailo B, El-Sohemy A, Haddad PS, Arora P, Benzaied F, Karmali M, Badawi A. *Vitamins D, C, and E in the prevention of type 2 diabetes mellitus: modulation of inflammation and oxidative stress.* Biologics. 2011;5:7-19. Epub 2011 Jan 19.
Comment: Support for micronutrients, employed as a novel preventive measure for T2DM.
================================
Boucher BJ. Vitamin D insufficiency and diabetes risks. *Curr Drug Targets.* 2011 Jan;12(1):61-87.
Vitamin D insufficiency and diabetes risks.
Comment: Vitamin D(2/3) supplementation is cheap but whether some non-hypercalcemia-inducing analogue may prove safer has not yet been addressed at the population level.

Romieu I, Trenga C. *Diet and obstructive lung diseases* Epidemiol Rev. 2001;23(2):268-87
Comment: Emphasises five fruits and vegetables/day.

==================================

Li Y, Schellhorn HE. *New developments and novel therapeutic perspectives for vitamin C.* J Nutr. 2007 Oct;137(10):2171-84.
Comment: Encouraging results in vitamin C therapy.

==================================

Jacob RA, Sotoudeh G. *Vitamin C function and status in chronic disease.* Nutr Clin Care. 2002 Mar-Apr;5(2):66-74.
Comment: More appreciation of Vitamin C nutriture possibly being more important for people with certain diseases or conditions.

==================================

Portugal CC, da Encarnação TG, Socodato R, Moreira SR, Brudzewsky D, Ambrósio AF, Paes-de-Carvalho R. *Nitric oxide modulates sodium vitamin C transporter 2 (SVCT-2) protein expression via protein kinase G (PKG) and nuclear factor-κB (NF-κB).* J Biol Chem. 2012 Feb 3;287(6):3860-72. Epub 2011 Oct 31.
Comment: Nitric Oxide finely controls and shows importance of vitamin C access to cultured retinal cells and neural tissue
==================================

May JM. *"The SLC23 family of ascorbate transporters: ensuring that you get and keep your daily dose of vitamin C."* Br. J. Pharmacol. 2011 Dec;164(7):1793-801. doi: 10.1111/j.1476-5381.2011.01350.x.
Comment: The ascorbate transporters SVCT1 and SVCT2 shown to be vital to survival shown by genetically re-engineering mice.
==================================

Lau LI, Chiou SH, Liu CJ, Yen MY, Wei YH. "*The effect of photo-oxidative stress and inflammatory cytokine on complement factor H expression in retinal pigment epithelial cells.*" Invest Ophthalmol Vis Sci. 2011 Aug 29;52(9):6832-41.
Comment: These results provide a potential novel treatment strategy for age-related macular degeneration.
==================================
Yin J, Thomas F, Lang JC, Chaum E. "Modulation of oxidative stress responses in the human retinal pigment epithelium following treatment with vitamin C." J Cell Physiol. 2011 Aug;226(8):2025-32. doi: 10.1002/jcp.22532
Comment: Ascorbate supplementation of 100-200 µM appears to strongly inhibit OS-induced activation of AP-1 in vitro, and may retard Macular Degeneration but pretreatment with higher levels of ascorbate conferred no additional advantage. Possibly the special vitamin C pumps keeping the retina well supplied negated the effect of pretreatment.
==================================
Cano M, Thimmalappula R, Fujihara M, Nagai N, Sporn M, Wang AL, Neufeld AH, Biswal S, Handa JT. *Cigarette smoking, oxidative stress, the anti-oxidant response through Nrf2 signaling, and Age-related Macular Degeneration.* Vision Res. 2010 Mar 31;50(7):652-64. Epub 2009 Aug 22.
Comment: Age-related "Macular Degeneration (AMD) is the leading cause of blindness among the elderly. Effective treatment is unavailable. Cigarette smoking is the strongest epidemiologic risk factor, but can these researchers explain why CardioRetinometry has shown dramatic reduction of retinal ischemia in a young female cigarette smoker within a year of abandoning the habit?
==================================

Hsu CC, Wang JJ. *L-ascorbic acid and alpha-tocopherol attenuates liver ischemia-reperfusion induced of cardiac function impairment.* Transplant Proc. 2012 May;44(4):933-6.
Comment: Vitamins C and E protected cardiac function by scavenging hydroxyl radical and reducing lipid peroxidation. Vitamin C showed better protection than vitamin E in rats.

==================================

Oishi K, Hagiwara S, Koga S, Kawabe S, Uno T, Iwasaka H,
Noguchi T. *The vitamin E derivative, EPC-K1, suppresses inflammation during hepatic ischemia-reperfusion injury and exerts hepatoprotective effects in rats.* J Surg Res. 2012 Jul;176(1):164-70. Epub 2011 Apr 28.
Comment. Little to add.

===

Oelze M, Knorr M, Kröller-Schön S, Kossmann S, Gottschlich A, Rümmler R, Schuff A, Daub S, Doppler C, Kleinert H, Gori T, Daiber A, Münzel T.
Chronic therapy with isosorbide-5-mononitrate causes endothelial dysfunction, oxidative stress, and a marked increase in vascular endothelin-1 expression. Eur Heart J. 2012 May 3.
Johannes Gutenberg University, 55131 Mainz, Germany.
Comment: Isosorbide-5-mononitrate toxicity to endothelial cells was countered by vitamin C and may suggest why mononitrates fail.

==================================

Giussani DA, Camm EJ, Niu Y, Richter HG, Blanco CE, Gott   schalk R, Blake EZ, Horder KA, Thakor AS, Hansell JA

Hansell JA, Kane AD, Wooding FB, Cross CM, Herrera EA. *Developmental programming of cardiovascular dysfunction by prenatal hypoxia and oxidative stress.* PLoS One. 2012;7(2):e31017. Epub 2012 Feb 13.
Abstract (Very abbreviated)
Comment: Fetal hypoxia is a common complication of pregnancy known to programme cardiac and endothelial dysfunction in the offspring in adult life. On day 6 of pregnancy, rats (n = 20 per group) were exposed to normoxia or hypoxia ± vitamin C. Maternal vitamin C prevented these effects.

================================

Fernández-Robredo P, Recalde S, Arnáiz G, Salinas-Alamán A, Sádaba LM, Moreno-Orduña M, García-Layana A. Effect of zeaxanthin and antioxidant supplementation on vascular endothelial growth factor (VEGF) expression in apolipoprotein-E deficient mice. Curr Eye Res. 2009 Jul;34(7):543-52.
Comment: Zeaxanthin and antioxidants may delay or reverse alterations in the retinal pigment epithelium and deposits in Bruch's membrane and reduced Vascular endothelial growth factor expression observed in apoE(-/-) mice.

================================

Kalariya NM, Ramana KV, Srivastava SK, van Kuijk FJ. *Genotoxic effects of carotenoid breakdown products in human retinal pigment epithelial cells.* Curr Eye Res. 2009 Sep;34(9):737-47.
Comment: The genotoxic effects of lutein (LBP) and beta-carotene breakdown products may be prevented by glutathione in retinal epithelial cells but DNA damage and cell death incurred by lutein breakdown products although prevented by N-acetylcysteine.
Maeda T, Maeda A, Matosky M, Okano K, Roos S, Tang Hosoya K, Nakamura G, Akanuma S, Tomi M,

Tachikawa M. *Dehydroascorbic acid uptake and intracellular ascorbic acid accumulation in cultured Müller glial cells (TR-MUL).* Neurochem Int. 2008 Jun;52(7):1351-7. Epub 2008 Feb 14.
Comment: Dehydroascorbate is taken up by facilitative glucose transporters, most likely GLUT1, and converted to AA in TR-MUL5 cells.
==================================
Rózanowski B, Burke J, Sarna T, Rózanowska M. *The pro-oxidant effects of interactions of ascorbate with photoexcited melanin fade away with aging of the retina.* Photochem Photobiol. 2008 May-Jun;84(3):658-70. Epub 2008 Feb 7.
Comment: Photoexcited melanin from retinal pigment epithelium induces photo-oxidation of ascorbate with concomitant generation of hydrogen peroxide. Age-dependent shift in the pathways with which ascorbate interacts in human retinal pigment epithelium were found. Ascorbate acted on oxidation pathways in the retinal pigment epithelium of the old. UV shorter than 340 nm wavelength was rapidly more damaging but still damaging at 600nm.
==================================
Drobek-Słowik M, Karczewicz D, Safranow K.*[The potential role of oxidative stress in the pathogenesis of the age-related macular degeneration (AMD)].* Postepy Hig Med Dosw (Online). 2007;61:28-37 Review.
Comment: Intensive oxygen metabolism, excess light, high polyunsaturated fatty acids, free radicals, oxidative stress are aggravated by lipofuscin increasing with age. Especially older than 65. Cigarettes smoking, obesity, blue light, bright irises all predispose. Naturally protective macular pigment is formed by dihydroxycarotenoids, lutein and zeaxanthin. The prereceptoral location of the macular pigment filters short-wavelength visible light.

Antioxidant carotenoids, vitamins C, E, carotenoids and zinc considered preventative.

=================================

Droy-Lefaix MT, Cluzel J, Menerath JM, Bonhomme B, Doly M. *Antioxidant effect of a Ginkgo biloba extract (EGb 761) on the retina.* Int J Tissue React. 1995;17(3):93-100.
Comment Ginkgo Biloba was shown by its general free-radical scavenger properties, to be usefully antioxidant, inhibiting retinal impairments observed after lipoperoxide release.

=================================

Mah E, Matos MD, Kawiecki D, Ballard K, Guo Y, Volek JS, Bruno RS. *Vitamin C status is related to proinflammatory responses and impaired vascular endothelial function in healthy, college-aged lean and obese men.* J Am Diet Assoc. 2011 May;111(5):737-43.
Comment. They conclude that more vitamin C might help prevent cardiovascular disease.

=================================

Charach G, George J, Roth A, Rogowski O, Wexler D, Sheps D, Grosskopf I, Weintraub M, Keren G, Rubinstein A. Baseline low-density lipoprotein cholesterol levels and outcome in patients with heart failure. Am J Cardiol. 2010 Jan 1;105(1):100-4.
Source: Department of Internal Medicine, Tel Aviv Sourasky Medical Center, Tel Aviv, Israel. drcharach@012.net.il

Comment: Heart failure increases in the Western world. Statins for primary and secondary prevention lower low-density cholesterol. LDL cholesterol as an adverse prognostic predictor in patients with advanced HF is controversial. The lowest LDL cholesterol levels had the highest mortality. Heart failure cases treated with statins had the worst prognosis.

====================================

Gurdasani D, Sjouke B, Tsimikas S, Hovingh GK, Luben RN, Wainwright NW, Pomilla C, Wareham NJ, Khaw KT, Boekholdt SM, Sandhu MS.
Lipoprotein(a) and Risk of Coronary, Cerebrovascular, and Peripheral Artery Disease: The EPIC-Norfolk Prospective Population Study. Arterioscler Thromb Vasc Biol. 2012 Oct 11. Source: Department of Public Health and Primary Care, Institute of Public Health, University of Cambridge, Cambridge, United Kingdom.
Comment: Lp(a) levels predicted peripheral arterial disease and coronary disease and was not improved by low-density lipoprotein cholesterol levels. This is a powerful vindication and confirmation of Pauling-Rath theory.

====================================

Galli F, Iuliano L. Do statins cause myopathy by lowering vitamin E levels? Med Hypotheses. 2010 Apr;74(4):707-9. Epub 2009 Nov 6.
Source: Faculty of Pharmacy, Department of Internal Medicine, Section of Applied Biochemistry and Nutritional Sciences, University of Perugia, Via del Giochetto, 06126 Perugia, Italy. f.galli@unipg.it
Comment: These researchers have become very interested in the suspected depletion of vitamin E by statins. This may at least in part be also linked to the muscle weakness and pain associated with this drug.

Xavier D, Devereaux PJ, Goyal A, Pais P, Yusuf S.

Polypharmacotherapy for primary prevention of cardiovascular disease. Indian Heart J. 2008 Mar-Apr;60(2 Suppl B):B29-33.
Source
Population Health Research Institute, Department of Medicine, McMaster University, Hamilton, Canada. denis@ccc.mcmaster.ca
This relatively old research highlights the cardiovascular problems of a vast and largely vegetarian population, significantly foregoing red meat.
==================================
Fischer T. A new possible strategy for prevention and preventive treatment of age-related macular degeneration resting on recent clinical and pathophysiological observations. Orv Hetil. 2009 Mar 15;150(11):503-12. [Article in Hungarian]
Comment: It is suggested that endothelial dysfunction is addressed by drugs with much emphasis on oxidative stress but not on vitamin C.
==================================
Nozue T, Yamamoto S, Tohyama S, Umezawa S, Kunishima T, Sato A, Miyake S, Takeyama Y, Morino Y, Yamauchi T, Muramatsu T, Hibi K, Sozu T, Michishita I; Kanagawa PTCA Conference Study Group Treatment with statin on atheroma regression evaluated by intravascular ultrasound with Virtual Histology (TRUTH Study): rationale and design. Circ J. 2009 Feb;73(2):352-5. Epub 2008 Dec 26.
Collaborators (39) Source
Division of Cardiology, Department of Internal Medicine, Yokohama Sakae Kyosai Hospital.
Comment. In order to evaluate regression of coronary artery plaque these researchers had to use gray-scale

intravascular ultrasound. Actual changes in coronary artery plaque composition produced by statin therapy could not be delineated. Why not use CardioRetinometry and SEE the ACTUAL plaque? We noted that arterial plaque regression is admitted. So why not an end point for treatment?

================================

J Am Pharm Assoc (2003). 2008 Nov-Dec;48(6):803-7. Riche DM, East HE, Priest HM. Practical management of dyslipidemia with elevated lipoprotein(a). J Am Pharm Assoc (2003). 2008 Nov-Dec;48(6):803-7. Source Schools of Pharmacy and Medicine, University of Mississippi, Jackson, MS, USA. driche@sop.umsmed.edu Comment: Niacin was used to reduce Lp(a). They conclude that Lp(a) is a secondary cardiovascular risk factor. It would appear to be more of a risk 'marker' according to Paling-Rath theory. Why didn't they use vitamin C?

================================

Reynolds TM, Mardani A, Twomey PJ, Wierzbickid AS. Targeted versus global approaches to the management of hypercholesterolaemia. J R Soc Promote Health. 2008 Sep;128(5):248-54. Source: Clinical Chemistry Dept, Queen's Hospital, Belvedere Road, Burton-on-Trent, Staffordshire DE13 0RB, UK., tim.reynolds@burtonh-tr.wmids.nhs.uk Comment: These authors claim that the role of statins in secondary prevention of cardiovascular disease is well established. It isn't. Much data has been published that is far from convincing and also much that is contradictory e.g., above, Gurdasani D, Sjouke B,

Tsimikas S, Hovingh GK, Luben RN, Wainwright NW, Pomilla C, Wareham NJ, Khaw KT, Boekholdt SM, Sandhu MS.
Lipoprotein(a) and Risk of Coronary, Cerebrovascular, and Peripheral Artery Disease: which supports the Pauling-Rath theory.
==================================
Petretta M, Costanzo P, Perrone-Filardi P, Chiariello M. Impact of gender in primary prevention of coronary heart disease with statin therapy: a meta-analysis.
Int J Cardiol. 2010 Jan 7;138(1):25-31. Epub 2008 Sep 14. SourceDepartment of Clinical Medicine, Immunological and Cardiovascular Sciences, Federico II University, Via S. Pansini 5 Naples 80131, Italy. petretta@unina.it
Comment: Much more reasonably these researchers admit that the role of statin therapy in primary prevention is still controversial, in particular for female gender. They conclude that statins do not appear to have a beneficial effect on total mortality for both men and women in primary prevention. CONCLUSIONS:
Our study showed that statin therapy reduced the risk of CHD events in men without prior cardiovascular disease, but not in women. Statins did not reduce the risk of total mortality both in men and women.
=========================
Mennickent C S, Bravo D M, Calvo M C, Avello L M.
[Pleiotropic effects of statins]. Rev Med Chil. 2008 Jun;136(6):775-82. Epub 2008 Aug 26. [Article in Spanish] Source Departamento de Farmacia, Facultad de Farmacia, Universidad de Concepción, Casilla 237, Concepción, Chile. smennick@udec.cl
Comment: Questionable conclusions are reached suggesting that elevated serum cholesterol, especially

the LDL fraction, is a major cause of coronary heart disease (CHD). VLDL cholesterol is a risk 'marker.'

==

Brody S. High-dose ascorbic acid increases intercourse frequency and improves mood: a randomized controlled clinical trial. Biol Psychiatry. 2002 Aug 15;52(4):371-4.

Source

Center for and the Psychosomatic and Psychobiological Research, University of Trier, Germany.

Comment: Ascorbic acid as they say, modulates catecholaminergic activity, decreases stress reactivity, approach anxiety and prolactin release, improves vascular function, and increases oxytocin release. It appears to increase intercourse and the differential benefit to noncohabitants suggests that a central activation or disinhibition, rather than peripheral mechanism may be responsible. (Other work suggests that it also increases fertility)

==

Kisic B, Miric D, Zoric L, Ilic A, Dragojevic I.
Antioxidant capacity of lenses with age-related cataract. Oxid Med Cell Longev. 2012;2012:467130. Epub 2012 Jan 29. Source: Institute of Biochemistry, Faculty of Medicine, 38220 Kosovska Mitrovica, Serbia. bojanabk2002@yahoo.com

Comment: They state that the immediate cause of the occurrence of cataract is unknown, but oxidative damage and effects of reactive oxygen species are considered important in its etiopathogenesis. The concentration ratio of redox couple DHA/AA is higher in lenses with mature cataract, where the measured concentration of AA was lower than in the incipient cataract.

Hettiarachchi NT, Boyle JP, Bauer CC, Dallas ML,

234

Pearson HA, Hara S, Gamper N, Peers C. Peroxynitrite mediates disruption of Ca2+ homeostasis by carbon monoxide via Ca2+ ATPase degradation. Antioxid Redox Signal. 2012 Sep 1;17(5):744-55. Epub 2012 Apr 5.
Source: Leeds Institute of Genetics, Health & Therapeutics, Faculties of Medicine and Health, University of Leeds, United Kingdom.

Abstract: AIM:
Sublethal carbon monoxide poisoning causes prolonged neurological damage involving oxidative stress. Given the central role of Ca(2+) homeostasis and its vulnerability to stress, we investigated whether CO disrupts neuronal Ca(2+) homeostasis.
RESULTS:
The antioxidant ascorbic acid inhibited effects of CO on Ca(2+) signaling, as did the peroxynitrite scavenger. *These researchers appear to be unaware of the Klenner flash oxidation of CO by IV ascorbate.*

INNOVATION:
The cellular basis of CO-induced neurotoxicity is currently unknown. Our findings provide the first data to suggest signaling pathways through which CO causes neurological damage, thereby opening up potential targets for therapeutic intervention.
Comment: CO stimulates formation of NO and reactive oxygen species which, via peroxynitrite formation, inhibit Ca(2+) extrusion via PMCA, leading to disruption of Ca(2+) signaling. We propose this contributes to the neurological damage associated with CO toxicity.
These researchers also appear to be unaware that Klenner found Carbon Monoxide to be flash oxidised by vitamin C.
=================================

235

Wray DW, Nishiyama SK, Harris RA, Zhao J, McDaniel J, Fjeldstad AS, Witman MA, Ives SJ, Barrett-O'Keefe Z, Richardson RS. Acute reversal of endothelial dysfunction in the elderly after antioxidant consumption. Hypertension. 2012 Apr;59(4):818-24. Epub 2012 Feb 21
Wray DW, Nishiyama SK, Harris RA, Zhao J, McDaniel J, Fjeldstad AS, Witman MA, Ives SJ, Barrett-O'Keefe Z, Richardson RS.
Source Geriatric Research, Education, and Clinical Center, Salt Lake City Veterans Affairs Medical Center, Salt Lake City, UT 84132, USA. walter.wray@hsc.utah.edu
Comment: As usual, honest statement of apparent facts such as aging being associated with a pro-oxidant state and a decline in endothelial function is not matched by an apparent awareness of the need for the specific naming of the type of vitamin E used. *The standard form used in studies is synthetic, rendering them useless studies.*
================================
Spangenberg T, Grahn H, van der Schalk H, Kuck KH.
[Paraquat poisoning. Case report and overview].
[Article in German] Med Klin Intensivmed Notfmed. 2012 May;107(4):270-4. Epub 2012 Jan 19.
Source II. Medizinische Abteilung/Kardiologie, Asklepios-Klinik St. Georg, Lohmühlenstr. 5, 20099, Hamburg, Germany. t.spangenberg@asklepios.com
Comment: Klenner would have given no other treatment than IV ascorbate.

================================
Stolle LB, Heidemann E, Bischoff-Mikkelsen M.
[Scurvy is not entirely a historical disease].
[Article in Danish]

236

Ugeskr Laeger. 2012 Feb 20;174(8):499-500.
[Scurvy is not entirely a historical disease].
[Article in Danish]
Source: Plastikkirurgisk Afdeling, Odense Universitetshospital, 5000 Odense, Denmark. stolle@ki.au.dk
Comment: As they say - Scurvy, lack of vitamin C, is a rare disease and is often called seafarers' disease. This case story describes a 36 year-old female patient with scurvy after a gastric bypass operation. Scurvy led to severed bullae on the skin, haemorrhagia and loose skin. After intensive care and a minor split skin graft she was discharged to a local hospital. Three months later she died of sepsis. Klenner would have said that insufficient vitamin C caused the sepsis.
====================================
Meena H, Pandey HK, Pandey P, Arya MC, Ahmed Z.
Indian J Pharmacol. 2012 Jan;44(1):114-7.
Evaluation of antioxidant activity of two important memory enhancing medicinal plants Baccopa monnieri and Centella asiatica. Indian J Pharmacol. 2012 Jan;44(1):114-7. Source Herbal Medicine Division, Defence Institute of Bio-Energy Research (DIBER), DRDO, Field Station, Pithoragarh-262501, Uttarakhand, India.
Comment: Free radicals or highly reactive oxygen species are capable of inducing oxidative damage to human body. Antioxidants terminate reactive species, reducing the disease risk. Baccopa monnieri and Centella asiatica are used to treat brain disorders in humans. Antioxidant activity was evaluated by measuring reducing ability, free radical scavenging activity. Regular use of Baccopa monnieri could be more helpful compared to Centella asiatica in treatment of neurological disorders caused by free radical damage.

Ig Sanita Pubbl. 2012 Jul-Aug;68(4):523-32.
[Benzene in soft drinks: a study in Florence (Italy)].
[Article in Italian]
Bonaccorsi G, Perico A, Colzi A, Bavazzano P, Di Giusto M, Lamberti I, Martino G, Puggelli F, Lorini C.
Source
Dipartimento di Sanità Pubblica, Università degli Studi di Firenze.
Comment: Two citrus fruit-based drinks were found to have benzene levels above the European limit for benzene in drinking water of 1 µg /L. Not all soft drink producers have eliminated benzoic acid from soft drinks as recommended by the European Commission. Benzene in trace amounts in all beverages suggests that migration of constituents of plastic packaging materials or air-borne contamination may be occurring.

=================================

Invited article: Current opinion | Published 3 February 2012, doi:10.4414/smw.2012.13515
Cite this as: Swiss Med Wkly. 2012;142:w13515
Statins: Have we found the Holy Grail? Raban Jeger, Thomas Dieterle Cardiology, University Hospital, Basel, Switzerland
Comment: In coronary artery disease, cardiovascular risk factors are the main targets for primary and secondary prevention. Statins prevent cardiovascular events in patients at risk. However, despite the proven efficacy and safety of statins, relevant side effects exist and should be considered when treating patients.
As they say - Lovastatin became the first commercially available statin in 1987, followed by simvastatin

pravastatin, atorvastatin, rosuvastatin, and pitavastatin (table 1) [3]. Cerivastatin had to be withdrawn from the market in 2001 due to side effects [4].Statins are competitive inhibitors of the 3-hydroxy-3-methylglutaryl-coenzyme A (HMG-CoA) reductase that is responsible for a rate-limiting step in cholesterol biosynthesis at the cellular level [5, 6]. By inhibiting the conversion of HMG-CoA to mevalonic acid, statins imitate the action of vitamin C.

================================

From the Wikipedia.
(Never used for serious research)
Cerivastatin (Baycol) was voluntarily withdrawn from the market worldwide in 2001, due to reports of fatal rhabdomyolysis. During post-marketing surveillance, 52 deaths were reported in patients using cerivastatin, mainly from rhabdomyolysis and its resultant renal failure. Risks were higher in patients using fibrates, mainly gemfibrozil (Lopid), and in patients using the highest (0.8 mg/day) dose of cerivastatin. Bayer A.G. added a contraindication for the concomitant use of cerivastatin and gemfibrozil to the package 18 months after the drug interaction was found. The frequency of deadly cases of rhabdomyolysis with cerivastatin was 16 to 80 times higher than with other statins. Another 385 nonfatal cases of rhabdomyolysis were reported. This put the risk of this (rare) complication at 5-10 times that of the other statins. Cerivastatin also induced myopathy in a dose-dependent manner when administered as monotherapy, but that was revealed only after Bayer was sued and unpublished company documents were opened.

================================

Shatzer AN, Espey MG, Chavez M, Tu H, Levine M, Cohen JI. Ascorbic Acid Kills Epstein-Barr Virus (EBV)

This put the risk of this (rare) complication at 5-10 times that of the other statins. Cerivastatin also induced myopathy in a dose-dependent manner when administered as monotherapy, but that was revealed only after Bayer was sued and unpublished company documents were opened.

==================================

Shatzer AN, Espey MG, Chavez M, Tu H, Levine M, Cohen JI. Ascorbic Acid Kills Epstein-Barr Virus (EBV) Positive Burkitt Lymphoma Cells and EBV Transformed B-Cells in Vitro, but not in Vivo. Leuk Lymphoma. 2012 Oct 16. [Epub ahead of print]

Comment: Confirmation of Cathcart's work in vivo regarding vitamin C killing Epstein-Barr virus and positive Burkitt lymphoma cells. They found it ineffective in mice that were suffering severe combined immunodeficiency.

Bibliography
Sugar and Diabetes:
Reiser S., et al. Blood lipids, lipoproteins, apoproteins and uric acid in men fed diets containing fructose or high amylase cornstarch. Am. J. Clin. Nutr. 1989; 49:832-9.

Eat less sugar. The Lancet Dec. 23 19089, 1538.

Brand-Miller, Janette C. Importance of glycaemic index in diabetes. Am J. Clin. Nutr. 1994. 747S-752S.

American Diabetes Assn. Clinical Practice Recommendations 1998. Position Statement: Nutrition recommendations and principles for people with Diabetes Mellitus. Diabetes Care, 1998: 21 (Supplement)

Apovian C.M. Sugar sweetened soft drinks, obesity, and Type 2 Diabetes. Jama Aug 2004 292(8) 978-979.

Cohen A.M. et al. Experimental models in Diabets.

Sugars in Nutrition, San Francisco Academic Press. 1974.
Yeap S K, Mohd Ali N, et al. Antihyperglycemic effects of fermented and nonfermented mung bean extracts on alloxan-induced-diabetic mice. J Biomed Biotechnol. 2012;2012:285430. doi: 10.1155/2012/285430. Epub 2012 Oct 3.

References

Abrahamson, E.M. , M.D., and A.W. Pezet, Body Mind and Sugar, Holt Reinhart, Winston, New York, NY, 1951.

Airola, Paavo, Every Woman's Book, Health Plus Publishers, Sherwood, Oregon, 1979.

Baker, Elizabeth and Dr. Elton Baker, The Uncook Book, Promotional Publishing, San Diego, CA, 1980.

Baker, Elizabeth and Dr. Elton Baker, The Un Diet Book, Promotional Publishing, San Diego, CA, 1984

Baker, Elizabeth, and Dr. Elton Baker, The Un Medical Book, Promotional Publications, San Diego, CA, 1997.

Baker, Elizabeth, Does the Bible Teach Nutrition?, Wine Press Publishing, Mukilteo, WA, 1997.

Baker, Elizabeth, The Un Medical Miracle: Oxygen, Promotional Publishing, San Diego, CA, 1986.

Balch, Phyllis, C.N.C., and James Balch, M.D., RX Prescription for Dietary Wellness, PAB Publishing, Inc, Grenfield, IN, 1992.

Balch, James, M.D., and Phyllis Balch, C.N.C., RX Prescription for Nutritional Healing, Avery Publishing Group, Inc. , Garden City Park, NY, 1990.

Becker, Robert, M.D., and Gary Selden, The Body Electric, William Morrow and Company, Inc., New York, NY, 1985.

Bland Jeffrey PhD., Vitamin C The Future Is Now. A HealthComm/Keats Publication. ISBN 0-87983-685-7

Bureau of Cardiovascular Research, The Doctor's Health Heart Formula, Alternative Medicine Updates, Marina del Rey, CA 1996.

Bush , Sydney, D.Opt, PhDhc, 700 Vitamin C Secrets, and 1,000 Not So Secret For Doctors Pp. 448, 1,889 listed entries. ISBN 978- 0-9566519-9-0 Pub. Direct POD/Lonsdale 2010.

Bush Sydney J. Rapid Response to Wong. eBritish Medical Journal 23rd July 2003.
Bush Sydney J. Rapid Response to Wong ebritishMedical Journal 26th Nov. 2003.

Bush Sydney J. (Subject of and Extract from) Pp 107-111 Ridiculous Dietary Allowance. An Open Challenge to the RDA for Vitamin C. Dr. S. Hickey PhD and Dr. H. Roberts PhD 2004 Pub Lulu. ISBN 1-4116-2221-9

Bush Sydney J. (Subject of and Extract from) Pp 46-49 Practicing Medicine Without A License - The Story of the Linus Pauling Therapy for Heart Disease. Dr. Owen Fonorow PhD. 2008 Pub Lulu. ISBN978-1-4357-1293-5

Bush Sydney J. (Subject of and extract from Thesis collaboration with Francis, Paul; Dept of Engineering Hull University for BSc. "Analysis of retinal Images For Health Care." for which Paul Francis gained 1st Class Honours BSc degree. 2007)

Carter, Mildred, Hand Reflexology, Parker Publishing Company, Inc., West Nyak, NY, 1975.

Cawood, Gayle, M.Ed., Janice McCall Failes, and Frank Cawood, The Prescription Encyclopedia, FC & A Publishing, Peachtree, GA, 1989.

Cheraskin, Emmanuel, MD., Dr. Marshall Ringsdorf, Jr., and Dr. Emily Sisley, The Vitamin C. Connection, Harper & Row Publishers, Inc., 1983.

Colgan, Michael, The Right Dose: Your Personal Vitamin Profile

Cummings, Stephen, MD, and Dana Ulman, MPh, Everybody's Guide to Homeopathic Medicines, G. Putnam's Sons, New York, NY. 1991.

Consumer's Guide to Prescription Drugs, Ed., Consumer's Guide, Publications International, 1991.

Davis, Adelle, Eat Right to Keep Fit, Penguin Group, New York, NY 1970

Davis, Adelle, Let's Get Well, The New American Library, New York, NY, 1972

Cheraskin, Emanuel, , Dr W. Marshall Ringsdorf Jr, and Dr Emily Sisley, The Vitamin C Connection, Harper and Rowe, New York, NY, 1984

Diamond, Harvey and Marilyn, Fit for Life, Warner Books, New York, NY. 1985

Dobelis, Inge, Ed. Reader's Digest, Magic and Medicine of Plants, Pleasantville , New York, 1988.

Douglas, William Campbell, MD, Second Opinion Publishing, Atlanta, GA, 1996.

Frank, Benjamin, and Philip Miele, Dr. Frank's No Aging Diet: Eat and Grow Younger, The Dial Press, New York, NY, 1976.

Goertzel Ted. PhD. Goertzel Ben PhD., Linus Pauling: A Life of Science & Politics. ISBN 0-465-00673-6

Gottfried, Sandra S, Biology Today, Mosby, St. Louis, 1993
Gregory, Dr. Scott, "Holistic Protocol for the Immune System"
Healthy Healing: An Alternative Healing Reference, Spillman Printing, Sacramento, CA, 1985.
Hickey (Steve PhD.) & Roberts (Hilary PhD) The Cancer Breakthrough ISBN 978 1-4303-2300-6

Hickey (Steve PhD.) & Roberts (Hilary PhD) Ridiculous Dietary Allowance Amazon. ISBN 9-781411 622210 0

Hickey (Steve PhD.) & Roberts (Hilary PhD) Ascorbate. The Science of Vitamin C. ISBN 1-4116-0724-4 Lulu. 2004

Hill, Napoleon with Clement Stone, Success Through a Positive Mental Attitude, Pocket Books, NY, NY, 1977, p 7.

Hoffer A. MD., PhD., FRCP. Orthomolecular Treatment for Schizophrenia Keats Good Health Guides ISBN 0 87983-910-4

Howell, Edward Dr, with research contribution by Maynard Murray MD, Enzyme Nutrition, Avery Publishing Groups, Inc.1985.

Hutchison, Michael, Mega Brain: New Tools and Techniques for Brain Growth and Mind Expansion, Beech Tree Books, New York, NY, 1987. ISBN 9-78034541032-0

Institute of Medicine. Dietary Reference Intakes for Vitamin C, E Selenium and Carotenoids, 2000. ISBN 0-309-06935-1

Jensen, Bernard PhD, Clinical Nutritionist, Arthritis, Rheumatism and Osteoporosis: An Effective Program for Correction Through Nutrition, Bernard Jensen Enterprises, Escondido, CA, 1986.

Jensen, Bernard DC, Nutritionist, Doctor Patient Handbook, Bernard Jensen Enterprises, ,Escondido, CA, 1984.

Jensen, Bernard, DC and Mark Hanson, D.C., Empty Harvest, Avery Publishing Group, Garden City, NY, 1990.

Jensen, Bernard, DC, Love, Sex and Nutrition, Paragon Press, Honesdale, PA,1988.
Jensen, Bernard, D.C, Co-authored with Sylvia Bell, Nutritionist, Tissue Cleansing Through Bowel Management, Bernard Jensen Enterprises, Escondido, CA, 1981.

Jensen, Bernard, D.C., Ph.D., The Science and Practice of Iridology, Volume I, Bernard Jensen Publishing, Escondido, CA, 1995.

Jensen, Bernard, D.C., Ph.D., Tissue Cleansing Through Bowel Management, Bernard Jensen Publishing, 1981, Pages 107 - 113.

Jensen, Bernard Jensen, with Anderson, Mark, Empty Harvest, Avery Publishing Group, Inc., , Garden City Park, New York, 1973, p 46

Kirschmann, Gayla and John Kirschmann, Nutrition Almanac, 4th Edition, McGraw-Hill, New York, NY, 1996. Pages 202 - 205

Klenner Frederick R. MD., FCCP. Clinical Guide To The Use Of Vitamin C (Abbreviated and summarized and annotated by Dr. Lendon H. Smith MD) Life

Sciences Press 1988 ISBN 0-943685-13-3
Kloss, Jethro, Back to Eden, Woodridge Press Publishing Company, Santa Barbara, CA 1975.

Kordich, Jay, The Juiceman's Power of Juicing, William Morrow and Company, Inc., New York, NY, 1992.

Leibert, Mary Ann, Soya for Health: A Definitive Medical Guide, Mary Ann Leibert Publisher, Larchmont, NY 1996.
Family Guide to Natural Medicine, Reader's Digest Association, Inc., Pleasantville, NY, 1993.

Levy Thomas E. MD., JD. Stop America's #1 Killer. Reversible Vitamin Deficiency Found to be Cause of ALL Coronary Heart Disease. 650 Scientific References. Livon Books. ISBN 0-9779520-0-2 Pub 2006

Levy Thomas E. MD., JD. Vitamin C, Infectious Diseases & Toxins – Curing the Incurable.1,200 Scientific references.ISBN 1-4010-6963-0

Lucas, Richard, Nature's Medicines, Universal Publishers, New York, NY, 1968

Mark, Vernon H,MD, FACS, with Jeffrey Mark M.Sc. Brain Power, Howton Mifflin, Boston, MA 1989.

Mason-Hunter, The Healthy Home,
        By Linda Mason Hunter

McFailes, and Frank Cawood, Encyclopedia of Top Secret Ways to Defeat "Old Age", FC & A Publishing, Peachtree,Ga.

Mindell, Earl, The Vitamin Bible, Warner Books, New York, NY, 1979.

Nautilus Press, Your Birthday Series, New York, 1990, p 48

Ody, Penelope, The Complete Medicinal Herbal, Dorling Kindersley, London, 1993.

Paps, Andreas. (The Vitamin E Factor)

Passwater, Richard A. Ph.D., The Super Nutrition, Pocket Books, New York, NY, 1991.

Passwater, Richard A, PhD, The New Super Nutrition: Your Guide to Super Helth and Vitality, Pocket Books, New York, NY, 1991.

Pauling, Linus, PhD, How to Live Longer and Feel Better, Avon Book, New York, NY, 1986.ISBN 0-380-70289-4 and Oregon State University Press ISBN 10 0-87071-096-6

Ravnskov Uffe. MD., PhD. The Cholesterol Myths. Exposing The Fallacy That Saturated Fat and Cholesterol Cause Heart Disease. ISBN 0-9670897-0-0 New Trends Pub. 2000.

Reynolds, Joshua, MD, with Robert Heller, MD, and Christine McGinn Rogerson, 20/20 Brain Power partners, LLC, Laguna Beach, CA, 2005.

Robinson, Adam, What Smart Students Know

Sardi, Bill, The Anti-Ageing Pill. Here & Now Books. ISBN 09805640-5-8

Sardi, Bill, How to Live 100 Years Without Growing Old. Hyaluronic Acid, Nature's Healing Agent. ISBN 0-9705640-6-6

Sardi, Bill, In Search of The World's Best Water. ISBN 0-9705640-9-0 Here & Now Books Pub. 2001

Schauss, Friedlander-Meyer and Meyer,. Eating for A's

Smith, Kathy with Susan Levin, Walkfit for a Better Body, Warner Books, New York, NY, 1994.

Shook, Edward,
Advanced Treatise in Herbology,
Tennyson, E.T., The Diet of Oxygen, Harvest Publishers, Jefferson City, MO, 1956.

The Holy Bible, King James Version, Oxford University Press, New York, NY, 1945.

Turska, William A., NMD, Aethozol
Technical Manual, Scandia Publishers, Poulsbo, WA , 1993

Wade, Carlson, M.D., Inner Cleansing, Parker Publishing, West Nyak, NY, 1983.

Walker, Norman, Fresh Vegetables and Fruit Juices

Walford, Roy, M.D., Maximum Life Span, Avon Books, New York, NY, 1983

Walker Martin J. MA. Dirty Medicine Slingshot Publications. London ISBN 0-9519646-0-7

Willix, Robert D Jr, M.D., Maximum Health, Angora, Inc., Baltimore MD, 1993, Introduction.

Winters, June, Poisons in Our Food, Crown Publishers, Inc, New York, NY, 1991, P 203.

Wright, Jonathan V., MD, Dr Wrigjt's guide to Healing With Nutrition, Keats Publishing Inc.,1984.

From the Mercola website
Supplements Industry has an Unmatched Safety Record

Durbin is still on the war path against supplements, despite the fact that recent investigations in the US and the UK have concluded that supplements and herbal remedies have a sterling safety record. The UK-based, international campaign group, the Alliance for Natural Health International (ANH-Intl) recently revealed data showing that compared to supplements, an individual is:

Around 900 times more likely to die from food poisoning

Nearly 300,000 times more likely to die from a preventable medical injury during a UK hospital stay, which is comparable to the individual risk of dying that active military face in Iraq or Afghanistan

Additionally, the data shows that *adverse reactions to pharmaceutical drugs* are:

62,000 times more likely to kill you than food supplements

7,750 times more likely to kill you than herbal remedies

The data, which was collected from official sources in the UK and EU, demonstrate that both food supplements and herbal remedies are in the 'super-safe' category of individual risk – meaning risk of death from their consumption is less than 1 in 10 million.

Similarly, the latest data from the U.S. National Poison Data System (2010 report) NO deaths were from laboratory studies of animals. The Sprague-Dawley breed of rat is an example of a much used model.

Unfortunately for the taxpayer hoping to benefit from such experimental use of animals to test drugs and to a much lesser extent, nutrients, these experiments have been doomed to irrelevancy by the discoveries of Montel-Hagen, Sitbon and Taylor, who discovered to their astonishment that the blood of mammalian species, always assumed to behave in the same way as that of humans, does not in fact do so. This discovery followed on that of May, Qu and Whitesell, who had discovered that the blood of humans could revive vitamin C and much faster than imagined.

Biphasic action of vitamin C.

Renal threshold in humans.

There are two phases in which vitamin C exists in the blood plasma. Let us say that the first is above what is called renal threshold and the second is below that level. Renal threshold is the level at which when the plasma level is falling due to excretion in the urine, perspiration, via the lungs or faeces, the kidneys will not allow the loss of further vitamin C into the urine. Pumps called glomerular pumps in the kidney, work on the first urinary filtrate, to extract valuable salts, and other metabolic essentials that the body cannot afford to lose. These are returned to the blood stream. Vitamin C is returned to the blood stream when the level would otherwise fall below 14mgs/litre of plasma. Doctors, when asked if a person might be suffering a shortage of vitamin C, are trained at medical school by professors of physiology to respond, that it is extremely unlikely as nobody suffers from scurvy in this country today. In this way people are encouraged to believe that the 'old fashioned' disease of scurvy, which killed thousands of seamen until the British Government ordered the supply of lime juice, had 'gone away." This is deceitful. People are just as vulnerable as ever.

If pressed by the patient with the question "What will happen if I have more vitamin C?" the doctor is trained to answer that the body will simply reach 'tissue saturation' and the 'excess' will be voided in the urine giving the person 'the most expensive urine in the street." The doctor must not mention that this will not deter him from drinking the vintage champagne his patient might never be able to afford in his lifetime.

If the patient persists and asks the doctor "Is there any actual danger in having too much vitamin C?" the doctor is trained to reply that there might be as the excess might be converted into oxalate that could cause kidney stones.

An informed patient can then ask the doctor how this can be possible when the good doctor has assured the patient that after tissue saturation has been reached, excess is voided? It leaves the question, if oxalic acid is now to be produced, where is the spare metabolic capacity to be found? By the doctor's definition, tissue saturation has been reached and he can find no answer. Ask why the starving rat still excretes urinary vitamin C and he will reply that you can't compare humans with rats. Ask then, why, rats are used for so many experiments? Ask the doctor if it has not been found that kidney stones are caused by an infection? The nanobacter – nano – because it is at the limit of visibility with an ordinary light microscope. And ask if he knows that, despite his fears, no oxalate type kidney stone has ever been found but all contain the nano bacteria. Could the rats know this? In 1946 Dr. W.J.McCormick published a paper in 1946 explaining that kidney stones are scurvy. "Lithogenesis and Hypovitaminosis," *Medical Record* 159:7, July) three years before my professor tried to persuade us that "excess vitamin C causes kidney stones!"

Above renal threshold the concentration of vitamin C in the plasma is very dependent on and responsible for many things - Hormone production, destruction of histamine, quenching of extremely dangerous, life shortening free radicals, conversion of vitamin C into hydrogen peroxide to fire as bullets into bacteria engulfed by phagocytic white cells patrolling the bloodstream seeking out pathogens before they can infect brain, teeth, lungs, heart or other organs. It seems that we just cannot have enough vitamin C! How quickly does the level fall from a maximum reached perhaps 30 minutes after taking a gram or two? The maximum level, according to the work of Hickey and Roberts, seems to decline by 50% every 30 minutes. So after peaking during the next three hours at say, 40 mgs/litre (28mgs above renal threshold of 14mgs) you will lose 14mgs of your 28mgs 'excess.' Over the next hour you would lose 7 and then 3.5 mgs until after two more hours you would be down to a sixteenth of that i.e. a quarter of a milligram above renal threshold. At this level you might catch somebody's cold and feel that vitamin C was not serving you well. Below renal threshold, the level falls at vastly different rates for different people depending on their alleles. One person might not succumb to scurvy on an exclusion diet for as long as three months if at all, and another might die suddenly of perhaps, an Infection that would not be linked to the deficiency. Pneumonia is the most likely and is cured by Liposomal ascorbate. (Alan Smith NZ) : Two of three polymorphic haptoglobin alleles (2-1 and 2-2) are linked to vulnerability to scurvy and the 1-1 type conferring resistance to the disease. (Vol. 2 may include this.)

I would say that in my best opinion, all puzzling sudden deaths are likely to be traceable to scurvy in some way. Conditions as far apart as pneumonia, blood poisoning, atrial fibrillation, influenza, colds aneurysm and coronary thrombosis and stroke are all likely to be sponsored by scurvy. Dr Klenner felt that most if not all sudden deaths in infants had their roots in scurvy.

Working towards a better understanding of antioxidant function, they state that Dynamic Flow restores human physiology to the condition of animals that synthesise their own vitamin C. Unfortunately, the work of May, Qu and Whitesell of 1995 followed by the aforementioned startling discovery of Montel-Hagen, Sitbon and Taylor published this month, April 2009 (the encyclopedia was first published in October 2010) may compel us to modify that view. It now appears that, at least below renal threshold (for it is a biphasic system and this is now what I am sure others must join me in suggesting for a reasonable modus operandi, because we agree that we see the continuous excretion of ascorbate as essential for a healthy urogenital system when we have spare) the blood can now be seen to be acting as a unitary organ maintaining a constant optimised ratio of ascorbate to dehydroascorbate for its continued desirable vitamin C excretion. As Montel-Hagen, Sitbon and Taylor say, in this most recent discovery not yet reported in the media for reasons we simply cannot understand although now nearly a month old, "it had always been assumed" that mammalian blood of all species behaved in the same way. But, as they point out, they found a 'dramatic' difference in that only in human's does erythroidal glutathione recycling of the monodehydroascorbate anion take place in the red cell's cytoplasm with return to the plasma of L-ascorbic acid. To add to the complexity of the dynamic flow model, May, Qu and Whitesell (a haematologist doctor with a sense of humour) found that, acting as a unitary organ, the erythroidal component of whole blood is able to re-reduce the entire monodehydro-ascorbate anion of the system for conserving vitamin C and to reprocess the entire plasma complement every three minutes.

In addition it appears that there are further differences which require investigation. Of course this means that, rather than being at a disadvantage compared with the animals and, given the intelligence to seek out and use vitamin C optimally to provide a constant 1,000 times more than we need in our gut as a reservoir, it seems that we can meet and overcome challenges that would kill the animals that are rate limited in their production. Indeed, the reason why not all are killed by new strains of infections for which nobody possesses antibodies, may be that a limited number of extremely blessed individuals, enjoying the best of both worlds, can make extra vitamin C whilst drawing on that provided by a sensible diet chosen for a rainy day. The popular saying "Everything in moderation," is then seen as suicidal, showing little understanding of the facts or a sentence of death for a child if it is the dictum of doctors or parents. Klenner would have none of that. May J.M, Qu Z.C, Whitesell R.R. *Ascorbic acid recycling enhances the antioxidant reserve of human erythrocytes.* <u>Biochemistry.</u> 1995 Oct 3;34(39):12721-8. See dynamic flow. Absorption Intestinal: Authorities Richard C Rose and John X. Wilson have new views on this describing the small intestinal wall as quite leaky to small monovalent electrolytes and not passing ascorbate to any significant extent. They believe that the advantage of this to the organism in times of lack of vitamin C in the diet is that the amount in the blood does not leak the other way – back into the gut to add to the excreta. This would quickly result in scurvy and death. As they say however – there is a problem in having as they put it – a 'tight' (to ascorbic acid) gut wall. If the ascorbic acid can't diffuse from the blood into the intestinal chyme, it also cannot diffuse from dietary sources into the blood. The same is true for sugars and amino acids and many other water soluble nutrients. Quite excitingly they continue to describe how "a rather elaborate protein has been genetically dispatched into the brush border membrane of the enterocyte (absorptive cell). This specific protein is the entire key to how vitamin C is absorbed in animal species that have lost the capacity for absorption of it." Modestly they then continue with the blockbuster gem of information that had us wondering. "It thus appears that only those animal species which have a dietary need for ascorbic acid express high levels of Na^+ - ascorbate cotransport activity in the intestinal mucosa." That statement must surely have serious implications for experimentation on 'knockout' laboratory ODS animals in which the gamma L-Gulonolactone gene responsible for the final step of the conversion of blood glucose into vitamin C has been deleted. Obviously there can be no direct comparison with the dietary amounts found to be necessary for their survival compared with that of humans with a genetically adapted intestinal mucosa evolved over millions of years. It can now be seen that possibly most of all the vitamin C experiments that have been approved and trialed need to be repeated and even then – we could fall into the trap of believing that we know more than we do about this amazing substance. Further reference. Crane R.K. *Hypothesis for mechanism of intestinal active transport of sugars.* Fed Proc 1962. 21:891 See dynamic flow. (also Packer and Fuchs. 147)

KEMPNER W. Radical dietary treatment of hypertensive and arteriosclerotic vascular disease, heart and kidney disease, and vascular retinopathy. GP. 1954 Mar;9(3):71-92. Comment: With a Spartan rice diet Kempner photographed improvements in diabetic retinopathy over 50 years.

Dr Robert Cathcart's Table from His Famou 1981 Paper:

Vitamin C, Titrating to Bowel Tolerance, Anascorbemia and Acute Induced Scurvy; Medical Hypotheses. 1981 Nov;7(11):1359-76.

VITAMIN C, TITRATING TO BOWEL TOLERANCE, ANASCORBEMIA, AND ACUTE INDUCED SCURVY

TABLE I - USUAL BOWEL TOLERANCE DOSES

CONDITION	GRAMS ASCORBIC ACID PER 24 HRS	DOSES PER 24 HOURS
Normal	4 – 15	4 – 6
mild cold	30 – 60	6 – 10
severe cold	60 – 100+	8 – 15
Influenza	100 – 150	8 – 20
ECHO, Coxsackievirus	100 – 150	8 – 20
Mononucleosis	150 – 200+	12 – 25
viral pneumonia	100 – 200+	12 – 25
hay fever, asthma	15 – 50	4 – 8
Environmental and food allergy	0.5 – 50	4 - 8
burn, injury, surgery	25 - 150+	6 - 20
Anxiety and other mild stresses	15 - 25	4 - 6
cancer	15 – 100	4 - 15
ankylosing spondylitis	15 – 100	4 - 15
Reiter's syndrome	15 – 60	4 - 10
acute anterior uveitis	30 – 100	4 - 15
rheumatoid arthritis	15 – 100	4 - 15
bacterial infections	30 - 200+	10 - 25
infectious hepatitis	30 – 100	6 - 15
candidiasis	15 - 200+	6 – 25

Dr. Constance Tsao's table.

Food	Serving	Vitamin C (mg)
Acerola juice	3/ 4 cup (6 oz)	6595
Guavas	4 medium	672
Currants	1 cup	671
Guava sauce (cooked)	1/ 2 cup	405
Pineapple	1 cup	280
Grapefruit, Red or Pink	1 large	247
Grapefruit, White	1 large	206
Peaches, sliced	1 cup	200
Sweet red pepper	1/2 cup, raw chopped	141
Strawberries	1 cup, sliced	123
Strawberries	1 cup, whole	82
Orange juice	3/4 cup (6 fl oz)	75
Orange	1 medium	70
Grapefruit juice	3/4 cup (6 ounces)	60
Broccoli	1/2 cup, cooked	58
Grapefruit	1/2 medium	44
Potato	1 medium, baked	26
Tomato	1 medium	23

End Notes: The Wikipedia entry for Dr. F. Mason Sones claims wrongly, that he was the first to perform X-Ray Coronary Angiography. This was first performed by Dr. G. C. Willis. In Montreal in Attempts to correct this like attempts to achieve listing of CardioRetinometry in the Wikipedia have been fiercely opposed, presumably by pharmacy 'editors,' resulting in a lifetime ban on Sydney Bush for his efforts to see justice done. (Serial Arteriography in Atherosclerosis G.C. Willis, A.W. Light, W.S. Cow. Canad. M.A.J Dec 1954, Vol71, pp 562-568.)
Anemia:

Whilst not specifically an eye disease unless retinal and papillary anemia are noted vitamin C greatly improves the uptake of iron from food.

From the Wikipedia Chemistry Encyclopedia   – CardioRetinometry   [Headed for several years by a note that it is being considered for deletion, presumably by unhappy pharmacists and Bush being barred from editing!.]

"CardioRetinometry: Is a new science. It is the rapid assessment of the changing health of the cardiovascular system by retinal image comparisons from fundus cameras. Very small differences between such images can be almost impossible to detect except by enlargement and precise superimposition on the monitor screen for rapid alternation and comparison. The smallest variations in arterial health are manifested by the inspection of these time lapse images to become plainly visible. Particles of cholesterol can be seen gradually disappearing and disappear when nutritional supplementation is accepted into the diet. They reappear when good nutrition is lost. In young people more fruit improves the blood vessels, re-establishing blood flow. Almost closed vessels reopen. The retina darkens as blood supply is restored. Many formerly mysterious ocular diseases might now be readily explained.

Only good diagrammatic three dimensional illustrations properly convey the theory and haemodynamics of cholesterol deposition in the retinal vasculature. The new science lends itself to the study of the viscoelasticity of blood, and it rheological properties which can now be observed impacting in vessels.

The principles of the new science of CardioRetinometry were discovered in the clinic of Optometrist Sydney J Bush late in 1999 following the installation of the then first of the electronic fundus cameras in 1998. The search for microscopic displacements of blood vessels within the optic nerve head which might signify the onset of primary open angle glaucoma, led to the discovery of changes within the arteries which coincided with supplementation of the diet with vitamin C. The author had read the recent patents and theories of Linus Pauling PhD and cardiologist Matthias Rath MD. They had established for their US patent (and published in a paper in Medical Hypotheses) that vitamin C is a surrogate for Lipoprotein alpha. The author coined the term Circadian Atheroma to describe the daily (24 hourly) inflow and outflow of cholesterol in and out of the arterial endothelium. This third form of very low density cholesterol, not much found in animals, serves as a 'puncture' repair for Man and higher primates when collagen cannot be made quickly enough to repair arterial damage due to stretching and compression with pulse waves. During rest and sleep the arterial damage is made good in a rate limited system. Excessive wear with insufficient repair then leads to heart disease. Marathon runners' deaths are explained in this way. Excessive exercise is revealed by CardioRetinometry as the cause, possibly aggravated by lack of 'hyper' nutrition to compensate.

Nutritional Prophylactic and Therapeutic CardioRetinometry make possible prevention and reversal of arterial disease using nothing toxic. The new science will allow rapid assessments of research successes and failures in the quest for perfect arterial health and, correspondingly, life extension.

The latter therapeutic form is only available legally in the UK to physicians without a signed medical request to the optometrist. The former prophylactic form can be practised by Optometrists without restriction and is available to most people. Results with hundreds of subjects have yielded a pattern of irrefutable benefits to the cardiovascular system shown by arterial clearance and actual reductions of adverse changes in the calibre and shape of blood vessels, previously portending serious disease.

CardioRetinometry is expected to quickly become the principal and definitive method of assessment of arterial health. It has already proved itself in the first informal studies to show every indication of being the most effective system of preventive medicine with the achievement of rapid and extremely accurate observations of blood vessel changes. It is expected to show when stroke and heart attack risk have been reduced to a degree never before imagined possible. Heart attack and most strokes should become rare. CardioRetinometry has already demonstrated changes in the morphology of the retinal veins corresponding with partial blockage by cholesterol. Currently the received medical wisdom is that cholesterol does not deposit in veins. This is now seen to be untrue.

The originator of CardioRetinometry made this claim in the electronic British Medical Journal of 23rd July 2004 in a rapid response to a paper on the changes in retinal vasculature proving to be predictive of hypertension. Prof T.Y. Wong was challenged in that letter, again by the originator of CardioRetinometry, Optometrist Sydney J Bush. He followed this claim with another letter in the eBMJ Rapid Responses to Wong of 26th November 2004 partly because no physician had challenged his statements. In those letters he redefined scurvy as existing in ephemeral, easily diagnosable and chronic sub-clinical, easily missed forms. The latter is what has been proving fatal in the causation of now easily detectable and reversible blood vessel disease seen and recorded in the retina. This remains true at the date of entering this submission in the encyclopaedia.

The name CardioRetinometry was coined because the retina is being measured directly as a surrogate for heart. In reverse, the name would have been RetinoCardiometry, clearly inappropriate for eye examination. The differential in blood pressures between heart and eye make the microscopic retinal changes correspond with far greater changes in the coronary arteries where stretching and compression also are maximal compared with the minimal pressures

in the retina. This assists in establishing the system as a hypersensitive diagnostic."
Sydney J Bush PhD.hc. DOpt. (IOSc. London)

Latest
As we went to press new evidence came to hand from results almost too fresh to publish, based on research by Dr. Owen Fonorow of the Vitamin C Foundation. He wished to settle the argument about the relative absorption rates and amounts of vitamin C from its ascorbic acid and sodium ascorbate sources. To his surprise he was able to produce convincing evidence that ascorbic acid is absorbed from the stomach (in health) much more strongly than from the sodium salt. He measured his blood glucose before and after self administration of approx 4.5 grams of ascorbic acid and 5.0 grams of sodium ascorbate for equivalence. This cannot be taken to mean that in sickness the vitamin is not absorbed much more actively from a greater length of the intestine. The loss of the bowel intolerance' effect to larger doses is believed to be due its stronger absorption with none reaching the colon to 'draw' water osmotically into the intestine to force an evacuation.
There is clearly a great deal more to learn about absorption.

A very new report from Israel

Tali Burstyn-Cohen's team responded to our enquiry confirming that in December 2012, in mice, protein S was found to be vital to the circadian phagocytosis function of the retinal pigment cells in their role protecting the epithelial photoreceptors. We believe that since we know that Vitamin C is intrinsic to phagocytosis, a strong link is to be expected. Mice produce the human equivalent of 20 grams of ascorbate daily.

Saturated fats

On Tuesday, June 15, 2010, the proposed 2010 *Dietary Guidelines* were released by USDA and HHS recommending even more stringent reductions in animal fats and cholesterol than all previous guidelines (1980-2005). The *Dietary Guidelines Advisory Committee Report, 2010,* recommended that Americans reduce saturated fat intake from 10 to 7 percent of calories and continued to demonize dietary fats and animal foods rich in saturated fat such as egg yolks, butter, whole milk, cheese, and red meat. Dr. Eric B. Rimm, Associate Professor of Medicine, Harvard Medical School; Associate Professor of Epidemiology and Nutrition, Harvard School of Public Health, questioned what he called the "artificial limit" on dietary fat in the U.S. Dietary Guidelines. Whilst Dr Rimm was concerned with the apparent untruths in the official position, he ignored the massive evidence from the Masai that there is no harm in low carbohydrate diets, and was supported by Dr. Walter C. Willett, Chairman, Department of Nutrition, Harvard School of Public Health, who agreed with Dr. Eric Rimm, his Harvard associate.

Appendix (3)
From Dr Bush's "700 Vitamin C Secrets"
a personal experience,
Was it a coincidence? A bilateral event within 24 hrs in both eyes?

Vitreous
"I generally caution against high doses of B2 whilst the jury is out. In my opinion the known effect of lowering the viscosity of the vitreous might destabilize the vitreous gel, leading to excessive mobility of the organ particularly with fast Left and Right eye movements, leading to traction and detachment of the vitreo-papillary attachments."

This might precipitate 'tobacco dust' episodes and peripheral retinal tearing manifesting as flashes of light with rapid eye movement, easily seen in the dark. In such cases the previously described source of retinal detachment is irrelevant for, in the relatively avascular ora serrata, there is little risk of developing tortuosity without major retinal blood vessels." Ref: Hofmann H, Schmut O (1975) Albrecht Von Graefes Arch Klin Exp Ophthalmol. 1975;194(4 Suppl):277-81." "The influence of riboflavin on vitreous homogenate" reported "Sunlight causes a decrease of viscosity of a mixture of riboflavin and ox vitreous homogenate while without riboflavin no reaction can be observed."

Appendix (4)
As we go to press
A new discovery has been made that threatens to invalidate much of Western medicine.

H3O2

Apparently this is the new 'cellular' water found in cells which had always been assumed to be H2O.
It is believed to have electromagnetic properties assisting in between articulating surfaces in joints.

'Energised' water assumes this form

We are accustomed to hearing of 'Heavy Water' in atomic energy production so should it surprise us?

Does it mean that the preparation of Homeopathic remedies involved the creation of this new water?

What are the implications for Western medicine if Homeopathic remedies are found, after all, to possess properties vital to our physiology?

We await more information

Appendix 5
As we go to press

Morgellon's disease!
From illegal ChemTrails
(U.N. Agenda 21 – depopulation)

Another new informal discovery has been made that threatens to invalidate much of Western medicine.

Coloursafe bleach in the bath with Alfalfa tablets
Both internally and extrenally.
The good news came with John Hammell's report as President of the International Associates For Health Freedom (IAHF)
http://www.youtube.com/watch?v=12uwwIWYiQo
Apparently the parasites exit the body rapidly.

Blank for notes

Blank for Notes

Over for Subject Index

Absorption 29, 69, 79, 101, 108, 114, 115, 146, 165, 168, 171, 258, 266,
Absorption, Bacterial 72,
Accommodation 98, 174, 176,
Acetyl L-Carnitine 127,
Acetyl Carnosine (n-acetyl –L-carnosine) 29, 116, 120, 126,
Acetyl Choline 117,
Acetylcysteine (N-acetylcysteine) 227,
Acidophilus 77,
Adenosine triphosphate (ATP) 63,
Adrenal (all) 109, 110, 113, 129, 142, 143, 144,
Adrenals and DHEA 109,
Adrenalin 109, 211,
Adverse Reactions 9, 41, 42, 69, 70, 164, 207, 252,
Aerobic Metabolism 63, 93,
Aethozol System 62, 64, 65, 249,
AIDS 66,
Alanine 114,
Albuminuria 103,
Alcohol 40, 81, 120, 169, 171, 215
Aldehyde Scavenging 29,
Alfalfa, Morgellon's Disease Cure 270,
Alfa-mint tea 60,
Alloxan, 181,
Alpha GPC 113, 117,
Alpha ketoglutarate. 63,
Alpha Lipoic Acid 102, 121, 127, 172, 173,
Alum 42,
Aluminium 69, 87, (Aluminum)

Amaurosis 145,

Amino Acid Cysteine 48, 50,

Amino   Acid   Glycine   11,   195,

Amino Acid L-Lysine 10, 11, 50, 97, 104, 114, 121, 124, 128, 171, 172, 188, 195, 196,

Amino Acid Proline 11, 195,

Amino Acid Taurine 48, 50,

Amnesia, 9,

Amylase 181, 241,

Anascorbemia 72, 125, 199, 260,

Anaerobic glycolysis 62, 63,

Aneurysm 14, 38, 163, 189, 191, 195, 256,

Angina 51,

Animals Producing Vitamin C 38, 44, 45, 47, 51, 71, 73, 74, 75, 155, 200, 256, 257, 258, 263,

Aniridia 177,

Anisometropia 176,

Ankylosing Spondylitis 99, 260,

Anopsia 177,

Anshel, Dr Jeffrey OD. And Ocular Nutrition Society 32,

Antacids 76, 87,

Antibiotics 50, 120, 143, 177, 179, 180, 207,

Antibodies 55, 75, 257,

Antidiabetic effects 181,

Antihistamine 30, 81, 120, 162, 177, 179, 183, 197,

Antihistamine (Vitamin C as natural) 81, 119, 120, 162, 177, 179, 183, 197,

Antiinflammatory 92, 114, 103, 113, 222,

Anti-inflammatory effects of vitamin C 222, 223,
Antioxidants 12, 27, 29, 31, 40, 43, 49, 62, 73,
75, 99, 101, 102, 105, 107, 108, 111, 114,
116, 123, 124, 133, 135, 138, 139, 144, 150,
157, 159, 161, 166, 167, 175, 178, 180, 181,
    187, 192, 196, 199, 204, 206, 210, 213, 214, 218,
222, 227, 229, 234, 235, 236, 237, 256, 257,
Antioxidant status 40, 43, 164, 181, 204, 224, 229, 236,
257,
Antiperspirants 87
Antistress formula 123,
Anxiety 234, 260
Apathy and scurvy 36, 83,
Aperient 115,
Apparently Healthy People, Gambling with lives 204,
Appendicitis 143,
Appendix (appendicectomy) 60, 143,
Aqueous 28, 29, 37, 108, 116, 178, 195, 198,
Arc Eye 177,
Arginine (L-Arginine) 101, 127,
Argyll Robertson Pupil 177,
ARMD 133, 135,
Arnica Montana 92,
Arteries and Disease 8, 10, 11, 12, 13, 14, 16, 19,
23, 26, 27, 29, 30, 35, 36, 42, 43, 44, 55,
71, 101, 103, 112, 132, 143, 146, 147,
158, 162, 163, 164, 168, 170, 171, 173,
189, 190, 191, 192, 194, 195, 196, 197,
199, 200, 206, 211, 217, 222, 230, 231,
232, 233, 238, 259, 262, 263, 264, 265,

Arteriolar Reflex 11, 13, 14, 29, 35, 112, 132, 147, 196, 211,

Arterioles 11, 217,

Arteriosclerosis 28, 29, 55, 146, 189, 190, 192, 190, 194, 198, 199, 262, 206, 222, 230, 259, 262,

Ascorbate 28, 32, 48, 58, 64, 71, 73, 74, 85, 95, 100, 105, 114, 117, 136, 137, 141, 143, 150, 153, 155, 160, 169, 170, 171, 175, 176, 177, 178, 179, 180, 182, 183, 184, 185, 187, 195, 197, 200, 202, 210, 211, 212, 213, 214, 224, 225, 228, 235, 236, 246, 256, 257, 258, 266,

Ascorbate cotransport 258,

Ascorbic acid 66, 71, 74, 75, 105, 108, 151, 155, 159, 160, 161, 162, 179, 180, 183, 184, 198, 209, 210, 212, 213, 215, 226, 228, 234, 235, 239, 240, 257, 258,

Ascorbic Acid Absorption (Fonorow) 266,

Ascorbic Acid Absorption 29, 258, 266,

Ascorbic acid inhibits effects of CO on Ca(2+) signaling 235,

Asiaticoside 114,

Aspartame 169,

Aspartate, 114,

Aspirin 6, 18, 92, 97,

Astaxanthin 116

Asthma 214, 260

Atherogenesis 36, 198,

Atherolysis 21, 29, 111, 146,

Atheroma 12, 36, 37, 38, 112, 146, 192194, 211, 231, 263,

Atheroma Genetic Countermeasure 37, 38, 200,

Atheroma Metabolic Countermeasure 37, 200,

Atherosclerosis 28, 29, 55, 146, 189, 190, 192, 190, 194, 198, 199, 262, 206, 222, 230, 259, 262,

ATP 63, 235,

Atrial fibrillation 18, 256,

Atrophic changes 112, 133

Atrophy (Iris) 189, 191,

Atrophy (Muscle) 90, 93,

Atrophy (Optic nerve) 125, 178,

Ayuverdic medicine 181,

Azadirachta indica 181,

Bacterial Infections 30, 120, 161, 178, 179, 183, 260,

Babizhayev MA (and cataract) 29,

BassenKornweig syndrome 151, 186, 188

BBC (British Broadcasting Corporation.) 9, 15,

Bentonite, 60,

Benzoic acid 42, 238,

Beta carotene 67, 202, 203, 227,

Bietti and Glaucoma; Rome University Eye Clinic 28, 125, 141, 142, 143, 154,

Bifurcations 42, 183,

Bioavailability 48, 96, 101, 107, 116, 203,

Bioflavonoids 99, 141, 210,

Biological Age 55, 99,

Biomarkers (Aging) 55,

Bioprine 114,

Bisphenol Plastic Containers 220,

Biosynthesis of Vitamin C 155,

Bleeding gums 8,

Blepharitis 30, 178,

Blepharochalasis 178,

Blood (Peroxide injection) 67,
Blood (Phagocytosis) 255,
Blood (Poisoning) 256,
Blood (Pressure) 18, 76, 114, 127, 164, 195, 197,
Blood (Reducing power of) 257,
Blood (Retina and) 263)
Blood (Scurvy related conditions) 256,
Blood (Sealant function) 37,
Blood (Stickiness/ viscoelasticity of) 115, 263,
Blood (Stream) 5, 12, 64, 65, 192, 201,
Blood (Sugar intolerance) 80, 180,
Blood (Supply) 12,
Blood (Thinning) 18,
Blood (Thrombolysis and Pycnogenols) 105,
Blood (Thyroid test) 149,
Blood (Type "O" and fat metabolism) 80,
Blood (Unitary organ action) 74, 257,
Blood (Vessel integrity and) 117, 136, 137, 196, 205, 211, 212,
Blood (Warm blooded animals) 90,
Blood (Flow and Pycnogenols) 105,
Bone Health 87,
Bowels 50, 51, 58, 71, 72, 78. 83, 85, 91, 92, 119, 121, 126, 136, 137, 148, 180, 182, 184, 187, 188, 247,
Bowel effect 72,
Bowel (Aspirin effect on) 92,
Bowel (Enema) 59, 60,
Bowel (Health) 77,
Bowel (Tolerance - Intolerance) 48, 72, 121, 126, 136, 137, 148, 180, 182, 184, 186, 187, 188, 260,

Bowel (White willow effect) 92,
Brahmoside and Brahminoside 114,
British Broadcasting Corporation and Vitamin C. 11, 17,
Brush border membrane 258,
Bumetanide powerful 'loop' diuretic 7,
Burning eyes feeling 62, 151,
Burning mouth syndrome 103,
Burns 100, 179, 260
Caffeine 42, 81, 113, 114, 115,
Calcium 14, 49, 87, 88, 114, 115, 148, 165, 168. 200,
Calcium and Chocolate 87, 88,
Calcium transport and PMCA 235,
Camphor conflict with homeopathy 92,
Canal of Schlemm 28, 143, 155,
Cancer 6, 9, 23, 41, 51, 57, 61, 62, 63, 64, 66, 67, 69, 76, 78, 80, 81, 82, 83, 94, 102, 109, 110, 127, 150, 164, 166, 167, 203, 205, 209, 210, 212, 212, 245, 260,
Cancer (Anaerobic cells and) 62, 63,
Cancer (Ascorbate, ascorbic acid and) 209, 210, 212, 245, 260,
Cancer (Beta Carotene and; The Finnish farce) 203,
Cancer (Causes) 57, 62
Cancer (Cell death) 62,
Cancer (Chaparral and) 82,
Cancer (Chondroitin sulphate and reduced) 51,
Cancer (CoEnzyme Q10 and) 81,
Cancer (Coleus Forskolii and) 127,
Cancer (DHEA and) 109,
Cancer (Enstrom, Morishige-Murata findings) 209

Cancer (Estrogenic factors) 66,
Cancer (Everything in moderation and) 164,
Cancer (Facial Acne drugs and) 150,
Cancer (Fish & Chips and) 165, 166,
Cancer (Flaxseed oil and) 78
Cancer (Food) 41, 42,
Cancer (Green tea and) 102,
Cancer (Laughter and) 94,
Cancer (Ozone therapy) 66,
Cancer (Pau d'Arco and) 83,
Cancer (Pauling, Linus, and wife Helen) 209
Cancer (Peroxide and) 66,
Cancer (Perricone and) 51,
Cancer (Pharmaceuticals causing) 41,
Cancer (Phenacetin and) 6,
Cancer (Polyunsaturates and) 165, 166, 205,
Cancer (Prevention) 76,
Cancer (Stimulated by Vitamin C?) 62, 63,
Cancer (Sugar and) 80,
Cancer (Vitamin E and) 76, 205,
Cancer (Warburg and) 57,
Cancer (Wheatgrass juice and) 61
Cancer (X-Ray caused) 23,
Canderelle 169,,
Carbon dioxide 57, 153, 177,
Carbon Monoxide and Ca2+ 235,
Carbon Monoxide and Flash Oxidation 161, 235,
Carbon Monoxide and Neurotoxicity 235,
CardioRetinometry® 4, 7, 9, 21, 22, 27, 30, 33, 39, 43,
56, 71, 99, 111, 112, 113, 120, 121, 122, 123, 128, 132,

Cataract (Vitamin B2) 147,
Cataract (Zeaxanthin and) 139,
Catechin (+)-catechin (-)-Catechin 102, 114, 234,
Catecholaminergic effects and ascorbic acid 234,
Cathcart Dr. Robert MD 31, 73, 151, 174, 188, 208, 240, 260,
Celandine infusion 118, 149,
Central serous retinopathy 29, 146, 178,
Cerivastatin 239,
Cerebro-Spinal Fluid Pressure and Cerebro-Retinal Atheroma 112,
Cerebrovascular disorders 116, 230, 233,
Chalazion 178,
Chaparral 82
Chlorinating Activity 159,
Chlorine 93, 95, 167,
Chocolate 80, 88. 101,
Chlorophyll 61, 67, 78, 79,
Chocolate and Calcium 87, 88,
Cholesterol 11, 12, 13, 19, 36, 37, 41, 55, 86, 104, 111, 158, 161, 168, 169, 192, 194, 196, 197, 198, 199, 200, 207, 223, 229, 230, 232, 233, 234, 239, 249, 262, 263, 265, 267,
Cholesterol. Very Low Density 14, 38, 196, 232,
Cholesterol, home use monitor 162,
Chondroitin Sulfate 51, 89,
Chorioretinal inflammation 179,
Choroidal haemorhage 179,
Chromium 102, 128
Chronological Age 55,

Conjunctivitis (U/V) 179,
Conjunctivitis (Viral) 179,
Conjunctivitis, (Welders') 179,
Corey (Lazarou, Pomeranz and) 6, 164,
Corneal Neovascularisation 179,
Corneal Ulcer 30, 100, 150, 179,
Coronary (Heart - all) 6, 9, 11, 12, 13, 15, 16, 17, 18,
20, 22, 23, 26, 30, 34, 35, 36, 37, 39, 44, 45, 47, 48, 49,
50, 51, 52, 53, 54, 55, 82, 84, 85, 94, 101, 109, 111,
117, 121, 122, 123, 132, 133, 136, 143, 149, 163, 164,
165, 170, 172, 173, 191, 192, 197, 198, 199, 200, 205,
206, 207, 208, 212, 216, 217, 218 222, 226, 229, 230,
231, 232, 233, 234, 238, 243, 244, 248, 249, 255, 259,
262, 264, 265
Coronary angiography, 17, 262,
Coronary arterial plaque regression by statins 231,
232,
Coronary bypass 16, 143, 200,
Coronary Heart Disease 6, 10, 11, 12, 14, 16, 17, 19,
20, 22, 23, 26, 30, 35, 35, 36, 37, 39, 43, 44, 54, 55,
103, 109, 170, 191, 192, 197, 198, 208, 212, 229, 230,
231, 232, 233, 234, 238, 244, 248, 249, 259,
Coronary Thrombosis 13, 15, 18, 23, 29, 39, 97, 136,
163, 164, 207, 256,
Corruption 8, 9, 13, 15, 17, 19, 30, 162, 193,
Corrupt Medical Archive 155,
Corticosterone 109,
Cortisol 110, 113, 118, 144,
Cosmopolitan University, 33,
Cottage cheese 78,

Cotton wool spots 189, 191, 194,
Creosote Bush Tea 82,
Culpepper 83,
Curcumin 105, 128, 148,
Cutaenous Biology, 214,
Cyclamate 169,
Dacryoadenitis 180,
Davis Adelle 88, 120, 123, 141, 142, 143, 144, 145, 146,
147, 149, 150, 205, 244, 245,
Dehydroepiandrosterone (DHEA) 109,
Dehydroascorbic acid 74, 89, 160, 228, 256,
Demography 27
Deodorants 87,
Depletion-Repletion Studies 202,
Dermatitis 180,
Detached Retina 28, 29, 139, 145, 146, 148, 186, 194,
217,
Detoxosode 93,
DHAA 89,
DHEA 109,
Digestion 51, 75, 76, 87,
Diabetes 30, 41, 136, 158, 166, 180, 181, 182, 223,
241,
Diabetes Type 2 30, 112, 166, 182, 223, 241.
Diabetic Retinopathy. 30, 117, 180, 190, 191.
Diethylstilbesterol (teratongenicity – monsters) 6,
Dihydroxycarotenoids 229,
Dihydroxy vitamin D3 181,
Dimethylaminoethanol 113, 117.

Dirty Medicine (Martin J. Walker) essential reading 200,

DMAE 113, 117,

DMSO CARE! Topical use only 92, 120,

Dr. Nourish 57, 68,

Dr. Balance 57, 83

Dr. Cleanse 57, 58,

Dr. Oxygen 57, 60,

Drinks 61, 68, 80, 169, 238, 241.

Drinks, Decaffeinated 81,

Drusen 182, 185, 194.

Dry Eye, 28, 119, 177, 183, 187,

Dry Macular Degeneration, 27, 139, (See Macular)

Dynamic flow and vitamin C 258,

Dynamic Flow 73, 74, 75, 256, 257, 258, 259.

Dystrophy, 182.

Ectropion, 182.

EGCG 102,

Electromagnetic 'Cellular' Water 269,

Emotional blindness 152,

Emu Oil 92,

Endothelial dysfunction 103, 226, 227, 231, 236.

Enemas 59, 83,

Ensheathment of arterioles falsely taught 11, 35, 132, 196.

Enstrom James 9, 214,

Enterocytes 258,

Entropion 182,

Environmental 29, 43, 98,

Enzymes 16, 55. 75, 76, 79, 81, 87, 91, 127, 146, 155, 164, 171, 207, 239, 246.
Epic-Norfolk Lipoprotein and CHD study 230,
Epigallocatechin-3-gallate (EGCG) Green Tea. 87, 102, 128, 167, 210.
Epiphora 182,
Episcleritis 28,
Erythroidal Glutathione Recycling 73, 74, 161, 100, 257,
Erythroidal Recycling Only In Humans 73, 257,
Etiopathogenesis 234,
Excreta 258,
Exercise 18, 40, 47, 51, 52, 53, 60, 93, 94, 95, 140, 147, 216, 264.
Exercises, eye (Orthoptics is omitted) 140, 147,
Exophthalmos 182,
Expensive urine 37, 135, 254,
Exudative retinopathy 182,
Eye Drops 29, 34, 119, 120, 126, 149,
FADH2 63,
Fats 12, 80, 101, 145, 167, 192, 196, 267,
FDA 6, 41, 43, 96, 176, 221, 252,
Feverfew 92, 107, 115,
Fertilizer 39, 41, 50, 69,
Fibrillation 256,
Finnish Beta Carotene Study and Cancer Debacle 203,
Firmoss Huperzia serrata 115,
Flavoneglycoside 102,
Floaters 140, 182, 187,
Flour (Bleached) 41, 51, 80,

Flour (Soya) 12, 192.
Flour, Whole grain 42, 101,
Fluoride 93,
Folic Acid 88,
Fonorow Dr. Owen, 20, 22, 34, 73, 174, 244, 266,
Food, 77, Acidophilus See Acidophilus.
Food, Allergy 260,
Food, And Cancer 41, 51, 61,
Food, And Soya source of Daidzein 69,
Food, And Soya source of Genistein 69,
Food, Adulteration 41, 43, 53,
Food, Choices, 12, 40, 41, 43, 45
Food, Choices and Life Expectancy 54,
Food, Dr. Wiley's statement before FDA CEO: 41,
Food, Dreadful mistakes 12,
Food, Fast 12,
Food Frequency Questionnaires 136,
Food, Goitrogenic 69,
Food, IQ and, 12,
Food, Hemagglutinin clot promoting 69,
Food, Life without 62,
Food, Low fat 12,
Food, Microwaves and 70,
Food, Natto, Tempo, Miso types, Soy sauce 69, 161,
Food, Not protected 43,
Food, Organic – see organic food.
Food, Plastic packaging and 70, 220, 238,
Food, Poisons in, 41, 42, 171, 249, 251,
Food, Preserved 41,
Food, Preventing mineral 49, 68, 69, 73,

Food, Processed 41, 67, 79, 198,
Food, Raw, 40,
Food, Restaurant 41,
Food, Raw 40
Food, Retinal 164,
Food, Sexual development and 67,
Food, Soya 67,
Food, Soya restriction 69,
Food, Supplementation 65,
Food, Vitamin C Loss, 44,
Formaldehyde 169,
Formic acid, 169,
Free Radicals 12, 17, 31, 54, 62, 123, 148, 156, 158, 159, 160, 161, 180, 192, 228, 236, 237, 255,
Fructose 168, 241,
Fuchs, Jurgen 212,
Fungi 57,
Furosemide diuretic 7,
Gamma L-Gulono Lactone Gene 155, 258,
Gemfibrozil 239,
Germanium 129, 144, 145
Genocidal RDA for Vitamin C 156,
G6PD see Glucose-6-Phosphate 214,
Genotoxic effects of lutein 227,
Gifford-Jones W. MD., (Pen-name of Dr Walker) 4, 20, 31,
Ginkgolide B 102, 115, 121, 127, 140, 172, 229,
Glaucoma 22, 25, 28, 33. 34, 35, 112, 114, 117, 121, 125, 127, 128, 129, 136, 141, 142, 143, 144, 145, 147, 178. 182, 185, 189, 190, 191, 192, 217, 263,

Glaucoma, Optic Nerve Atrophy 125, 178,
Glaucoma (Primary Open Angle) 28, 125, 136,
142, 143, 185, 263,
Glaucoma: See entries for Bietti and Virno.
Glaucoma and stress, 128, 129, 141, 142, 143, 144,
147,
Glomerular pumps 253
Gluconic DMG 88,
Glucosamine 89, 172,
Glucosidase (Alpha) 181,
Glucose ascorbate antagonism theory (Ely) 169,
Glucose to ascorbate, 155,
Glucose 63, 80, 88, 110, 155, 160, 168, 169, 181, 200,
209, 214, 222, 228, 258, 266,
Glucose-6-Phosphate Dehydrogenase (Deficiency)
214,
Glucose transporter (GLUT -ascorbate) 160, 200, 209,
213, 224, 228, 258, 259,
GLUT see above.
GLUT 1 - Transporter missing invalidates mouse
research. 200.
Glutamate, 114,
Glutaryl-coenzyme 239,
Glutathione, 74, 257,
Glutathione   in   Retina   227,
Glycation 29, 103, 213
Glycation & Transglycation 29,
Glycerol and Vitamin E 48, 76, 171,
Glycolysis 62, 63,
Glycoside 102, 114,

Hedahl Dr. R. 4, 22, 34, 123, 128, 217,
Hemodialysis   103,
Hemaglutinin 69,
Herbs (See Selected Nutrient List) 6, 47, 59, 82, 83, 85,
89, 100, 118, 181
Herpes 182, 188,
Histamine 104, 151, 152, 153, 177, 197, 198, 199, 255,
Histaminosis 183
Histidine 114,
HMG Co-A reductase inhibition (Statins) 239,
Hoffer Abram 142, 153, 208, 246,
Holistic College 24, 245,
Holistic protocol 245,
Hollenhorst Microplaque 183,
Homeopathy 48, 50, 51, 92, 93, 149, 150, 244,
Homeopathy conflict with Tiger Balm. 92,
Homeopathy Veterinary 51,
Homeostasis 235,
Homozon 60, 67,
Honey 45, 80, 118, 120, 120, 206,
Hordeolum 30, 183,
Howerde, 212
Hunza, The Land of and Health of 132,
Huperzia Aqualupian 115,
Huperzia Carinat 115,
Huperzia 115,
Huperzia Serrata 115,
Huperzine 115,
Hydantoin-5-Acetic Acid 152, 177,
Hydrogen Peroxide 66, 68, 159, 228, 255,

Hydrogenated Oils 40,
Hypertension 36, 125, 236, 265,
Hypertensive Retinopathy 182, 183, 192, 259,
Hypochlorous Acid, 50 times more bactericidal 159,
Iatrogenic Deaths 5, 6, 9. 11, 13, 41, 43, 86, 164, 216, 239, 252, 256
Immune System 55, 57, 65, 69, 81, 84, 88, 89, 93, 104, 149, 160, 245,
Immunodeficiency Disease 214, 240,
Indigestion 76, 87,
Infantile scurvy 107, 182,
Insufflation 64, 65,
Intestinal Mucosa (absorption) 258, 259,
Intestinal wall "Leaky" 92, 258,
Intestinal wall "tight" to ascorbate 258,
Intestine Large 59, 114, 171, 258,
Intraluminal Plaque 10, 11, 13, 14, 17, 29, 35, 80, 122, 133, 147, 183, 200, 201, 223,
Intracellular ascorbic acid 228,
Intraocular Pressure see IOP 28, 112, 125, 142, 143, 154,
Intra-retinal stress 29, 146,
Intravascular Ultrasound 206,
IOP 33, 34, 112, 113, 126, 127, 128, 129, 141, 142, 143, 144, 154,
Iridencleisis 143,
Iridocyclitis 189, 191,
Iridology 247,
Iris atrophy 189, 191,
Iritis 150, 183,

Iron 103, 105, 107, 262,
Iron overload 103,
Irregular pupil 183,
Jaffe Dr. Russell and 130 gms /day 10,
Kale Kenton Unpublished Vitamin C research 155,
Kempner W. Cardiovascular & kidney disease 191, 259,
Keratitis 11, 100, 183,
Keratoconjunctivitis sicca 183,
Keratomycosis 184,
Keshan disease 203,
Key for Internet Images 242,
Kidney stones falsely threatened by physicians 254, 255,
Klenner Dr. Frederick MD., FCCP. and toxins 27,
Klenner Dr. Frederick 27, 31, 70, 72, 73, 75 155, 162, 174, 175, 184, 188, 208, 235, 236, 237, 247, 256, 257.
Kneble Dr. W. and brainwashed older doctors 113,
L-Arginine 101, 127,
Kryptopyrrole and Schizophrenia 153,
Lacrimal Gland 89, 184,
Lande & Sperry Revealing Cholesterol Fraud. 111,
Kritchevsky , David and cholesterol myth 207
Kritchevsky and false graphs of saturated fat consumption and Heart disease 207
Kryptopyyrole in Psychiatry. 153,
Laxative 59, 71, 78, 91, 164, 170, 169, 182,
Lazarou, (Pomeranz, and Corey) 100,000 Hospital Deaths per annum 6, 164
Leaky Gut 92,

Leprosy, 184,
Leucocyte (Function) 214,
Leishmaniasis 180,
L-gulono-lactone-gamma   oxygen   2-oxidoreductase,
gene, 155,
Life Expectancy 27, 44, 54,
Lifestream® Cholesterol monitor 161,
Linner and IOP in glaucoma 28,
Lipid 14, 29, 116, 195, 215, 223, 226, 232, 241,
Lipofuscin 228,
Lipoprotein 14, 36, 37, 199, 213, 221, 227,
229, 230, 232, 233, 241, 263,
Lipoprotein Alpha 14, 36, 37, 38, 199, 263,
Liposomal Glutathione 178,
Liposomal Vitamin C 178
Lipospheric (Reg) Vitamin C. 169,
Liver (all) 2, 6, 55, 66, 75, 89, 107, 126, 145, 155, 166,
171, 172, 177, 207, 226,
Liver damage / disease (main entries) 6, 9, 226,
L-Lysine 10, 11, 50, 97, 104, 114, 121, 124, 128, 171,
172, 188, 195, 196,
Lopid 239,
Lovastatin   238,
Lubricant 29,
Luminescent Therapy 68,
Lutein 28, 100, 101, 111, 114, 127, 133, 139, 175, 227,
229,
Lutein absorption 101,
Lycopene 101, 206,
Lymphocytes 55,

Medical Lies re Vitamins & Nutrients 252,
Medicine Orthomolecular 5, 15, 36, 154, 155, 188,
201, 246, 157, 189, 196, 201, 245, 252, 242, 248,
Medicine Toximolecular 5, 164,
Meta-analysis 164, 233,
Metabolic Capacity 254,
Metabolic Conversion of Histamine to harmless
metabolites 152,
Metabolic countermeasures 37, 200
Metabolic Essentials 253,
Metabolic Syndrome 103,
Metabolism 52, 63, 88, 94, 196, 203, 214, 222, 228,
253, 254,
Metabolites 109,
Methaqualone (addictive) 6,
Mevalonate 239,
Methyl alcohol, 169,
Microaneurysm 38, 189. 191,
Milk 45, 61, 70, 78, 88, 97, 104, 107, 121, 147, 165,
167, 168,
Mitochondria 21, 99, 103, 159,
Mitochondria (Biological clock) 21,
Molluscum contagiosum 184,
Montel-Hagen, Sitbon & Taylor 73, 74, 200, 209, 253,
256,
Monodehydro-ascorbic acid 74, 257.
Monounsaturated See Oils
Monovalent electrolytes 258,
Morgellon's Disease 270
Mouse model 174,

Mouse model unsatisfactory 200,
MPOD (macula pigment optical density) 175, 221,
MRSA 100, 179,
MS see Multiple sclerosis
Mucopolysacharide 51,
Muller Glial cells. 228,
Multiple Sclerosis 28, 103,
Muscle atrophy 90, 93,
Myeloperoxidase 159,
Myopathy 230, 239, 240,
N-Acetyl Cysteine 227,
Na+ ascorbate cotransport 258,
N-Acetyl Carnosine 29, 116, 120, 126,
N-Acetyl Cysteine 227,
NADH 63,
Nakanishi and MRSA cured by vitamin C. 100, 179,
Nasal shift 35,
Nasal obstructions 81,
Nascent Oxygen 67,
National Health Service (UK) 19, 123, 132, 158, 232,
National Institutes of Health. 15,
National Poison Data System (USA) 252,
Natto 69, 161,
Nausea 66, 148,
Neem tree 181,
Neovascularisation 133, 179, 189 190, 191,
Neovascularisation (Macula – wet) 133,
Neovascularisation (Cornea and) 179,
Neovascularisation (Glaucoma and) 190, 191,
Neovascularisation (Iris and) 190,

Neovascularisation (Optic disc) 189,
Neovascularisation (Perifoveal) 189
Neovascular (Secondary) glaucoma 189,
Neo-Zeaxanthin 101, 114,
Neurotoxicity and Carbon monoxide 235,
Niacin 105, 107, 142, 232,
Niacinamide 142,
NLM 15, 153,
Nomefensine (fatal hemolytic anemia) 6,
NSAIDs 92,
Nutrasweet 169,
Nyctalopia 184,

SELECTED NUTRIENT LIST

A-C Carbamide 129,
Agrimony 84,
Alfalfa 79, 270,
Alfa-Mint tea 60,
Almond milk 78, 88
Aloes 84,
Anti-inflammatories 92, 114, 222,
Apple juice 78,
Arnica Montana topical pain relief 92,
Avena Sativa 47.
Baccopa monnieri 237,
Betaine Hydrochloride 75,
Betaine Hydrochloride with Pepsin 76,
Bilberry 101, 116, 117, 126, 127, 140, 144,
Bilberry Eye Health Benefits 101, 116, 117, 126,
Blueberry leaves 84,

Blueberry root (Astringent) 84,
Blueberry vs Bilberry 116,
Blueberry Eye Health Benefits, 116,
Blue Flag tea 84
Blue green algae 79,
Blue Violet extract 84,
Broccoli 100 106, 170, 261,
Brussels Sprouts 100, 106,
Burdock Root Tea 83,
Butcher's Broom 47,
Carminative 115,
Carrot juice 79, 107,
Cascara Sagrada 59,
Cayenne 47, 48, 84, 107,
Cayenne (African) 84
Celery juice 79,
Centella asiatica 237,
Chickweed 84,
Chili powder 107,
Chlorophyll 61, 67, 78, 79,
Chrysamthemum (Feverfew) 92, 107, 115,
CoEnzyme Q10 16, 81, 121, 164, 171,
Collard Greens 100,
Coleus Forskolii (Prostate cancer warning) 127,
128, 129, Comfrey tea 84,
Crataegus (see Hawthorne) 47,
Cucumber juice, 79, 140,
Curcumin 105, 128, 148,
Dandelion root 84,
Dock Root Tea 83,

Neurotrophin Photomorphogen 129,
Oats 60,
Olive leaf extract 89,
Onions 101,
Oregon Grape 84,
Paprika 107,
Peas, 104,
Peripheral retinal degeneration, 146, 184,
Periwinkle Plant 116,
Pipsissewa 83
Proanthocyanidins 104,
Propolis (derived from herbs) 45, 88, 89,
Pycnogenols 105,
Pyrroloquinoline 128,
Red Clover Tea 83,
Red Wheat Kernels 61,
Rice milk 78,
Rock Rose 87
Romaine Lettuce 100,
Rosemary 47,
Sannie 47,
Saponins 47, 113,
Spinach 100, 101, 106, 111, 133, 140, 170, 175,
Spirulina Plankton 67, 78
St. John's Wort 83,
Tiger Balm topical pain relief 92,
Tomatoes 101, 106, 165,
Turmeric 105, 148,
Turnip Greens 100, 106,
Wheat Grass Juice 61, 67, 79,

White Willow 92.
Wintergreen 93,
Winter Squash, 106,
Yarrow 83,
Olive 80, 170,
Olive Leaf Extract, 89,
Olive Oil. (exception) 80, 165, 167,
Zucchini 100

END OF HERBS

RESUME SUBJECT INDEX

PDR Pocket Guide to Drugs 6,
Pepsin 76,
Peripheral Arterial Disease and Lipoprotein(a) 230,
Peroxidation (Lipid) 215, 216,
Peroxynitrite 235,
Pfeiffer Dr. Carl C. Vitamin C research 37,
Pharmacy 'controls' the media with advertising
wealth 8, 9, 130, 151, 156, 201, 211, 262,
Phenacetin (carcinogenic analgesic) 6,
Phenformin (Acidosis) 6,
Phlegm 58,
Phosphatidyl   serine   110,   113,   117,
Phosphorus 87, 107, 115,
Photographic Transmission of Evidence 4, 14, 30,
Photographic Proof 13, 36, 125, 132, 137, 138, 150,
Photographic Diagnosis of Incipient Retinal Disease
125, 138, 150, 185,
Photographic Proof or Retinopathy Reversal 191, 259,
Physician suppression of vitamin C (often revealed by
honest physicians) 8, 9, 15, 18, 30, 32, 33, 37, 97, 100,
134, 156, 158, 161, 162, 164, 174, 177, 180, 189, 192,
193, 194, 197, 199, 200, 203, 205, 208, 210, 212, 214,
225,
Physician training to suppress vitamin C 12, 32, 37,
253,
Phytonutrients 78, 108, 109, 112,
Placebo 51, 129, 130, 131, 141, 175, 176, 221,
Plaque (and Intraluminal) 10, 11, 12, 13, 14, 17, 29, 35,
80, 122, 133, 147, 183, 192, 200, 201, 223, 231, 232
Pneumonia 27, 256,

PubMed; Corrupted Archive of medical and nutritional information 130, 154, 157, 210, 221,

Puerh tea 181,

Pycnogenols 105,

Pyridoxine 105, 114,

Radiation 70, 116

Rath cardiologist Dr Matthias MD., 4, 11, 12, 14, 18, 21, 22, 30, 31, 35, 36, 37, 122, 157, 192, 194, 195, 197, 198, 199, 200, 208, 208, 209, 210, 211, 230, 232, 233, 263,

Raw Food 40, 44, 51, 67, 77, 79, 89, 105, 106, 107, 165, 170, 171, 261,

RDA Vitamin C. Determination Condemned for Mistakes 7, 203, 243

RDA For Vitamin C Childish Errors 203,

RDA For Vitamin C Genocidal, 7, 156, 200,

RDA For Vitamin E profit related 102, 205, 208,

RDAs (Various) 105, 115,

Red Eye 151, 185,

Red Meat 50, 68, 101, 231, 267,

Redox 213, 234, 235,

Refrigeration 44,

Regan, Ronald 102,

Renal disease 103,

Renal failure, 239,

Renal threshold 74, 166, 169, 253, 255, 257,

Re-reduction of Dehydroascorbate 73, 74, 160, 257,

Respiratory support 47, 64,

Respiratory burst (Phagocytosis) 159,

Respiratory chain 63,

Retina And Proof of Pauling/Rath Theory 11, 12, 22, 36, 212,
Retina And Sequential Imaging, 13, 30, 133, 262 ,263,
Retina And Tear Of, 28, 29, 30, 146,
Retina And Thrombosis of Vessels 29, 30, 146, 190, 191,
Retina And Tortuosity of vessels 29, 146,
Retina And U/V 178, 228,
Retina And Vitamin B2 147, 148
Retina And Vitamin Concentration Gradients 133,
Retinitis 30, 123, 146, 148, 150, 186,
Retinitis pigmentosa 150, 187, 186, 188,
Retinopathy 29, 30, 117, 146, 174, 178, 180, 182, 183, 187, 191, 259,
Retinopathy of Diabetes 30, 117, 180, 190, 191, 259,
Retinopathy, Exudative 176,
Retinopathy, Hypertensive, 176, 191,
Retinopathy, Serous 32, 146, 174,
Retinopathy 191, 257,
Retinopathy, Solar 187, 191, 257,
Retinoschisis 186,
Retrobulbar neuritis 28
Rhabdomyolysis 239,
Riboflavin (Vitamin B2) 114, 148, 225,
Rimland, Dr. Bernard 5
Rimm, Dr. 141, 267,
Risk Factor 37, 139, 148, 225, 232, 238,
Risk Marker 37,
Rice And Spartan Diet reduced diabetic 259,
River blindness 184, 186,

Scurvy, Medical Archive Education & Suppression, 15, 23, 32, 106, 122, 161, 197, 236, 253,

Scurvy, Ocular ischemia, 191

Scurvy, (Occult) 13, 16, 21, 179, 180,

Scurvy, not "gone away" 253,

Scurvy, Proof of conspiracy 130, 131, 212,

Scurvy, Proptosis 183,

Scurvy, Retinal detachment 187, 188,

Scurvy, Sudden Death 16, 255, 256,

Scurvy, Survival 122, 255, 256,

Scurvy, Unrecognised 13,

Selective Indexing 15,

Selenium 49, 102, 107, 121, 126, 148, 172, 203, 204, 206, 246,

Sesquiterpene 113,

Serine, 112, 116,

Serous retinopathy 29, 146, 178,

Shortness of Breath 81,

Similisan Line 119,

Sleep 40, 54, 96, 97, 110, 173, 198,

Smoke 138, 206, 214, 222, 223, 225,

Smoke, Second hand 62,

Soda Pop 45,

Sodium (alone or in combination) 32, 48, 64, 71, 105, 107, 137, 141, 143, 144, 153, 169, 170, 171, 179, 180, 183, 184,187, 210, 212, 224, 226,

Sodium (in ascorbate) (less than 15% of MWt.) 143, 171,

Soil 39, 60, 122,

Tissue Absorption 29,
Tissue Saturation 254,
Tobacco 40, 43,
Tobacco 'Dust' and Retinal Detachment 147, 268
Tocopherols See Vitamin E
Tocotrienols See Vitamin E
Tortuosity 29, 146, 186, 194, 268,
Toximolecular 5, 15, 164,
Toxoplasma 187,
Trabeculectomy 143,
Trabeculum 28, 112, 125, 141, 142, 143, 154, 183,
Trace minerals 21, 73,
Trichiasis 182,
Triterpene Glycoside (triterpenoid), 114,
Tunica intima 196,
Type 2 Diabetes 30, 166, 182, 223, 241,
Undernutrition 55,
Unexpressed Gulono Lactone gene 155,
Unified Theory Heart Disease 21, 22, 35, 37, 208,
Urethritis 187,
Useless Form of Vitamin E 49, 107, 210, 236, 265,
Uveitis 151, 183, 185, 187, 260,
Veins 12, 47, 65, 104, 189, 191, 192, 194, 217,
Venoms - Snake & Spider 27,
Vioxx 5, 6,
Vinpocetine 116,
Viral Infections 11, 178, 179, 182, 214, 260,
Virno and Glaucoma Rome University ye Clinic 28, 141, 154
Virus - ALL Virtually all pathogenic viruses 28, 31, 57, 58, 65, 70, 72, 77, 95, 100, 120, 159, 174, 178, 188, 239, 240, 260,
Viscoelasticity of blood 263,
Vitamin A 106, 126, 140, 150, 152, 184, 187, 204,
Vitamin B Deficiencies 151,
Vitamin B1 112, 170,
Vitamin B2 114, 187, 268,

Wong Prof. T.Y., Retinal disease researcher ignoring CardioRetinometry 36, 265,
Worms 217,
Wheat and Millers 41,
Wintergreen, Oil of. CARE! Topical use only. 93,
Wound healing 103,
Xanthelasma 187,
Xanthin alkaloids 114, 116, 127, 129, 133, 139, 144, 175, 176, 221, 227, 229,
Xerophthalmia 187,
X-Rays 17, 23,
Yaws 187
Yudkin John, Prof. "Sugar, Sweet, White, & Deadly." 168
Zeaxanthin 28, 101, 111, 116, 127, 129, 133, 139, 144, 175, 176, 221, 227, 229,
Zimeldine (Guillain Barr syndrome) 6,
Zinc 102, 105, 107, 128, 152, 229